The Gems of Genesis Wellness Blueprint

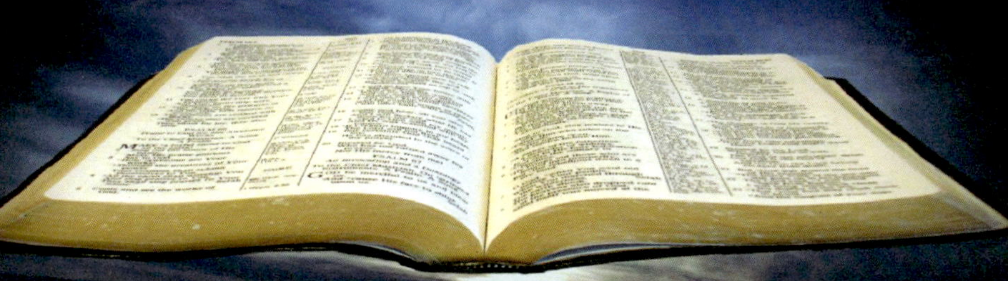

Sandy Stillwell

All scripture is taken from the New International Version (NIV) of the Bible unless otherwise indicated.

ISBN: 978-1-4951-8839-8

Authors Website: gemsofgenesis.com

Published by: Sandy Stillwell

Printed in USA

ACKNOWLEDGEMENTS

The Gems of Genesis Wellness Blueprint was developed as the Holy Spirit led me to many different books. My heart-felt gratitude is expressed for each author who poured out their life for their purpose. Each has illuminated a gem of wellness, and the ripple effect of their legacy lives on in these pages.

Say Good Night to Insomnia by Gregg D. Jacobs
Restful Insomnia by Sondra Kornblatt
Into the Light by William Campbell Douglass II, MD
Let there be Light by Darius Dinshah
Color Medicine by Charles Klotsche
Change Your Life With The Secret Power of Color by
Martin Kutternick and Colin G. Smith
Eat Right For (4) Your Type by James D'Adamo
Blood types, Body types and You by Dr. Joseph Christiano
Glorious Greens by Johnna Albi & Catherine Walthers
Whole Grains Every Day Every Way by Lorna Sass
Ripe, A Fresh Colorful Approach to Fruits and Vegetables by Cheryl Sternman Rule
Good Fats Cooking: Recipes for a flavor-Packed, Healthy Life by Franklin Becker
The Great Vegan Protein Book by Celine Steen and Tamasin Noyes
Flood Your Body with Oxygen by Ed McCabe
Bursting with Energy by Dr. Frank Shallenberger
The Forgiveness Project by Pastor Michael S. Barry
Law of Attraction by Michael J. Losier
Christ the Healer by F.F. Bosworth
Divine Healing Made Simple by Praying Medic
Heal the Sick by Charles and Frances Hunter
Understanding Your Dreams Now: Spiritual Dreams Interpretation by Doug Addison
Illustrated Dictionary of Dream Symbols by Dr. Joe Ibojie
How to Heal The Sick by Charles and Frances Hunter

A special thanks to my wonderful friends who proofread the earlier versions, and to my husband Jon, who supported every aspect of this dream.

A 'GEM' OF A REFLECTION FROM GENESIS

Rev. Ron Reaves, Retired Lutheran Pastor

Sandy Stillwell has skillfully mapped the wisdom and imagination of the biblical book of Genesis with her helpful direction for balance and wholeness for human life—God's crown of creation. Her cultivated skills as a health coach allows her to see the Creator's design as enabling renewal and restoration of life despite creaturely habits.

The wisdom of creation and nature are found by renewing energy in the cycles of light, color, and darkness. Creation holds innumerable miracles that point to the Creator's abiding love. In Genesis, we pull back the cosmic curtain a bit and wonder at the fine tuning of this blue and green planet, so wondrous and mysterious, that brings meaning within his magnificent design.

Stillwell's book is an informative read that shares vital information for health and wholeness to help you consider your own lifestyle, while marveling at the healing properties within the universe.

Janis Hutchinson, Bth, MA, award-winning author, health advocate

The Gems of Genesis Wellness Blueprint has broken new ground with Sandy Stillwell's inspirational encapsulation on how to renew energy, vitality and well-being using God's healing properties provided in the creation. She unveils the astounding impact on our health through the use of physical and soul nutrition, light-energy and color therapy in concert with one's genetic design, and correlates it with spiritual reflections on life-giving principles contained in the Bible. It is smart, well researched, and both physically and spiritually motivating. A much needed book for this age of rampant illnesses. A must read!

Pastor Dale L. Parkhurst

The Gems of Genesis is indeed filled with gems and insights of God's wonderful desire for every male and female to live a strong, healthy lifestyle. An eye-opener for me was: "Now you begin to arrive at the moment of truth—because what your mammal instinct intuitively tells you to eat, is the ultimate authority on health and nutrition. It is not what our minds tell us to eat but, rather, what our body truly directs." My eating habits were terrible and Sandy's book has enabled me to not only change my eating habits, but to see the value that proper nutrition plays in our lives, and why God designed the foods that He did for us. Sandy's thorough research and recommendations can help anyone make the changes necessary to live a long and healthy life as God has intended. "Thank you Sandy!"

The Rev. Jon R. Greenstone, Pastor,
Elias Evangelical Lutheran Church, Emmitsburg, Maryland

The Gems of Genesis presents inspiring insights that reveal God's plan for a completely healthy life. Sandy has a teaching gift that will enable the reader to find resilience and balance between the spiritual life and the physical being. She teaches practical principles for life-vitality through nutrition, and a healthy, vibrant self-image. She shares life-giving principles found in the "Gems of Genesis," God's treasured Word that reveals how to have a life filled with light and goodness. This comprehensive book motivates one to pursue health and wholeness in every area of life. Surely, you will be renewed in God's grace and love as you see this gem illuminated.

Anne James, Special Education Teacher and Tutor

The Gems of Genesis is a remarkable blueprint for healthy living, improving our physical and spiritual lives. Follow the precepts outlined in this comprehensive book, and you ***will*** become a healthier, happier, more fulfilled and complete person. This work deserves much recognition from experts and laymen alike.

Introduction

The book of Genesis reveals our wellness blueprint, embellished with rich symbolism and clues that guide us on the journey to optimum health. Here, in the intriguing literary masterpiece of Genesis, are twinkling jewels that revive and restore the core of our being as set forth by our Creative Designer, that blossoms into a three-part, body, soul, and spirit connection.

See how nutrition and fitness, combined with light, and color correlate with the principles of divine healing. The promise of the rainbow is not only to never again flood the earth, but to flood us with natural healing power.

Part 1 unveils the astounding impact of light, darkness, and color in our bodily systems, and the energy centers absorbed by our outer shell that harnesses electro-magnetic energy. The vital role of our etheric, or auric being (the energy field of the physical body) may not be well understood, since Western medical roots are grounded in the physical, mechanical plane. Yet, understanding this higher sphere can accelerate healing far beyond mechanical means. It's somewhat like the electrical components of our car or house. If a mechanical part isn't working, we first check to see if it's plugged in or if there are faulty electrical circuits which govern the mechanical. Likewise, when our mechanical parts (muscles, organs, tissues, bones, etc.) are dysfunctional or diseased, the root cause can often be restored in our etheric being, especially with color therapy, using light wave-lengths. Part one concludes with more recommendations to support your etheric being.

Part 2 presents your customized healthy lifestyle plan according to your blood, body type and emotional profile, including your nationality, age and gender. (Before launching into this section, it will be helpful if you know your blood-type.)

We'll explore the science of nutrition with a spiritual reflection of each food group derived from the scientific food pyramid. You can then implement the best foods, supplements, exercise and self-care specifically for your type. Beyond nutrition, we'll see how natural hormone replacement supports aging, and how exercise and breathing techniques invigorate us with oxygen enabling us to stay fully functional until our last breath.

Part 3 spotlights divine healing and prosperity in all ways. How do we actually become like Jesus in this dynamic way, since He commanded us to heal the sick and cast out spiritual darkness? How do we receive our own healing? While this may feel like a huge leap of faith, we can build our faith in practical ways using the science of the Law of Attraction with supporting scriptures. When faith comes as naturally and effortlessly to our spirit man, as seeing and hearing comes to our physical being, we'll lay our hands on the sick and they will absolutely rise!

Our destination is much more than being healthy, but rather, optimum health is the vehicle that propels us to soar to our highest calling. Each small step towards wholeness escorts us to full maturity, to become the light of Christ—piercing through the darkness!

Prologue
"Dust Thou Art..."

When I consider Your heavens, the work of Your fingers, The moon and the stars, which You have ordained; What is man that You take thought of him… (Psalm 8:3,4 NAS).

Have you ever wondered, what is dust? Dust is made of atmospheric debris, such as dead skin cells, dried feces, and the corpses of dust mites. What a humbling thought. (It makes me want to leave the dust bunnies under the bed.)

Yet, here's the beautiful part. Our Creator, the Master Recycler, has created man from this dust to be self-propelling, self-regulating, self-reproducing, and self-healing. Scientists are still discovering the mind-boggling capabilities of the supernatural human body, mind, and spirit.

Here's another grand thought about our meager existence. Since we are created from the atmospheric elements, we can restore our vitality by the wisdom of these very gems radiantly sparkling in the earth and gleaming in the sky.

Foreword –
"Our Symmetrical Universe"

In the beginning, God created …balance. The universe was created by polarities, opposites balancing each other. Likewise, optimal health is achieved by artfully using polarities in our lives. When we restore balance, we restore health. For instance, we commonly use polar forces for healing, such as heat to stimulate blood flow and cold to reduce inflammation (the elements of winter and summer). We'll see how we can harness polarities to create balance, and live healthy as we were designed.

A symmetrical universe of harmonious, complementary systems was established by balances and boundaries. Thus, there was light and darkness, day and night, morning and evening, winter and summer, sun and moon, land and water, plants and animals, and finally, Adam and Eve. Adam was formed from the earth and God breathed into him the breath of life.

As we connect with the elements of our foundation, we become like a well-balanced bicycle, riding fast and far from the natural energy within. Genesis is our handbook for superior maintenance. May we glorify Him in body and spirit as "His divine power has granted to us all things that pertain to life and godliness..." (2 Pet. 1:3 ESV). Certainly, this includes our health.

Let's now begin "in the beginning," where energy was generated from darkness and where day was separated from night, supporting our foundation of wellness by sleep and rest.

We'll explore how light energy powerfully radiates all life and gives birth to rainbow synergy which precisely heals all life. As we view this phenomenal light show of the natural and supernatural features of light, consider that the essence of our Creator is light.

Thus, when we read "God is light…" may the hairs on our skin rise to applaud in standing ovation; may our goose bumps become speed bumps to stop and praise Him. May we marvel with childlike wonder, as the Bible and science portray an impressive, harmonious masterpiece.

The heavens declare the glory of God;
the skies proclaim the work of his hands.

Day after day they pour forth speech;
night after night they reveal knowledge.

They have no speech, they use no words;
no sound is heard from them.

Yet their voice goes out into all the earth,
their words to the ends of the world.

In the heavens, God has pitched a tent for the sun.
It is like a bridegroom coming out of his chamber,
like a champion rejoicing to run his course.
It rises at one end of the heavens
and makes its circuit to the other;
nothing is deprived of its warmth. (Psalm 19: 1-6)

Now, let us harken to the voice of creation, receive the words of her healing speech, and become empowered by her knowledge longing to be revealed.

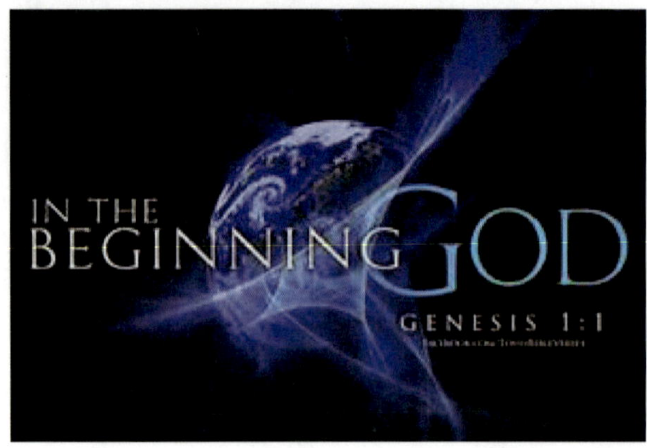

PART 1

Soul Nutrition
(etheric design)

We begin with soul life as our primary essence and dominance in this world. While the meaning of soul may have various theological implications, here I will use it in the basic biblical sense as one's *breath life, when "God breathed into Adam, and he became a living soul"* (Genesis 2:7).

For simplicity, let's consider the soul to be that which gives *life* to the physical body, in all of its complexity and dimensions. How wondrously we have been created, with our emotional etheric, or auric, layers (of the human energy field) intricately connected to our spiritual life.

Soul nutrition is the beginning of optimum health. As we synchronize with the natural circadian rhythm of the earth, we achieve better quality and quantity sleep, thereby recharging the human battery, and revitalizing our *circuits.* We'll explore how sunlight restores our total being with solar charging, and is the most powerful antibiotic and healing balm. Finally, we'll catch the amazing color lights of the rainbow that feed our etheric body, which then *heal* us physically and emotionally with specific light vibrations.

As a computer operates by an *electrical* source, so the human body and mind, the most sophisticated computer, are also empowered by an *electrical* source. Like physical electricity, the human *electrical components* and processes are not visible, except that the effects can be recognized in auric views.

In these chapters, biblical and scientific gems harmoniously support each other in proven healing modalities. We can experience health and healing far beyond mechanical means alone, by plugging into these amazing natural features of creation just as when we connect into an intimate relationship with our Creator, receiving His divine flow.

The foundation of Genesis is not only the beginning of humanity, but is our continual energy current empowering our whole being by revitalizing our electrical components. Health is measured not by *years,* but by our energy level. Let's see how we can plug into our Creator's master regenerating systems!

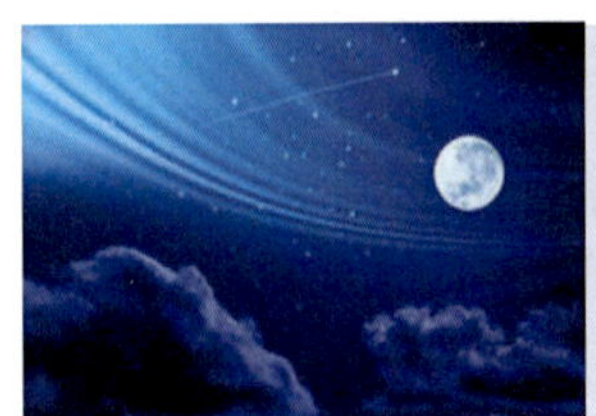

Chapter 1

The Healing Power of Night

In the beginning...darkness was over the surface of the deep...and he (God) separated the light from the darkness...and the darkness he called night. (Genesis 1:1,5)

Out of darkness the universe was born, and the Gems of Genesis adorned all life with the crown of health. Each element of creation bestows a profound impact on our well-being, with divine healing sparkling from unique angles in the day, night, seasons, land, water, oxygen, plants, animals, and the rainbow. As we synchronize with these natural healing modalities grounded in the science of man and the art of the Lord, we reap nature's amazing restoration. Let's begin this amazing journey through the first gem, *the night.*

Our supernatural design is to be perpetually self-regenerating and self-repairing. During deep sleep, our whole being is in a restorative marathon. Since the *night* (sleep) is the foundational *gem* for optimal health, the first consideration is improving sleep efficiency, a challenge for more than half of adults and many youths.

As a health coach, I was my first patient. Every few hours throughout the night, an alarm clock sounded in my head, leaving me wide awake. No sleep strategy seemed to help. After many zombie mornings, I realized that my sleeplessness was more than psychological. It was hormonal; and with hormonal therapy, I could finally sleep. Since hormone balance is essential for sleep and all bodily functions, a comprehensive evaluation with a *natural hormonal specialist* is foundational for optimum health.

For example, sleep impacts weight loss in many ways. Consider hormone communications somewhat like a traffic light, with a green light to *go*, a yellow to *slow*, or red to *stop*.

During deep sleep, fat burning hormones are predominately released, stimulating the metabolism, increasing energy, and balancing almost all bodily functions. Other hormones related to weight management are also secreted primarily during sleep. *Leptin* signals that you are full and to *stop* eating. "With the low-leptin levels…," says sleep researcher, Eve Van Cauter, "your body will crave carbohydrates even though you've had enough..." Then *Ghrelin* stimulates your appetite, driving you to eat more, leading to constant snacking and packing on the pounds. Sleep is essential to keep ghrelin from *growling* and allow *leptin* to *step in* and calm the raving beast. Additionally, high stress levels cause *Cortisol,* the stress hormone, to store fat. Stress absorbed during the day is carried into the night unless we release it prior to sleep. Once hormonally restored (if needed), there are other pieces to the puzzle of sleeping soundly.

After deep sleep *take-off*, we become *airborne* into deep sleep and then progressively into lighter sleep. This ensures our crucial *deep sleep* recovery mode first, no matter how much time we sleep.

Then, soaring into rejuvenating wonders, our temperature adjusts precisely for sleep. Body temperature is one of the most significant factors to achieving deep sleep, and our lifestyles can either *promote* or *prevent* a proper *temperature cycle.*

The good news is that your natural body temperature rhythm is *controllable.* While we may think that our body temperature remains the same continually, research reveals that it is closely linked to our level of activity throughout the day and night. When we're most active and alert, the body temperature rises; then as we grow sleepier, our temperature drops. Body temperature (B. T.) also rises when sunlight enters our eyes, and lowers as the sun sets. Of course, everyone has their own biological time clock. Night Owls function best at night because their body temperature peaks later in the day, while the Morning Larks' temperature peaks earlier.

Sleep specialist Dr. Gregg D. Jacob explains that less *variation* in B.T. rhythm throughout the day results in a flattened body temperature, with inactivity and sleeplessness. This may be because of less physical activity due to fatigue and delayed morning sunlight exposure to the eyes.

B.T. rhythm begins rising when we get out of bed, become active, and sunlight enters our eyes. Therefore, if you sleep a few hours later on the weekend, your B.T. is also delayed a few hours, and evening drowsiness is also delayed by the same amount of time, resulting in a too-high B.T. that feels like jet lag at bedtime.

Morning activity or exercise helps spike the B.T. earlier for greater peaks and dips in the day. While some are naturally owls, the closer we synchronize with the sun's pattern, the more energy we have throughout the day and in the night, for sleep. Therefore, rising earlier, at a fairly consistent time daily, maximizes the rise and fall of B.T.

During the *night,* our bodily systems also begin the night shift with *internal janitors.* Lymph fluid naturally drains by gravity through the lymph glands to release toxins stored up during the day. Much of our blood is directed to the muscles to replenish muscular energy and the immune system to work most effectively. Your *internal secretary* appears during dream time to review and organize new information you learned during the day to properly file and store in your memory. This enhances learning, and often leads to a fresh solution or outlook in the morning. As for measurable progress, we are actually slightly taller when we awake, due to gravitational depression. *How wonderfully we are created!*

In the night shift, the restoration operation begins. Our body runs on two twelve hour phases: the *catabolic stage* is from 6 a.m. to 6 p.m., and the *anabolic* is from 6 p.m. to 6 a.m. During the *catabolic* period, your body sacrifices by depleting one part of the body to give priority to a primary, such as the heart; thereby allowing temporary damage to one area to protect the priority member. Then, as we enter the *anabolic stage*, the body repairs the damage from the *catabolic* period. This process transpires especially during sleep through subtle energy fields that reach their maximum potential at the deeper levels of sleep. Adequate sleep is needed to repair the *daytime damage.* Chronic lack of sleep accelerates body deterioration, premature aging, and contributes to heart disease, diabetes, and obesity.

Another piece of the sleep puzzle is the psychological association of your sleep environment, specifically your bed and bedroom. It should be a strong cue for good sleep, rather than a *wrestling arena*. For instance, when we sit at our desk, we are mentally primed for work, or at the park, feelings of relaxation or play; so the bed must prompt us for sleep.

This queue is strengthened by reducing the time in bed to slightly more than the actual sleep time. If you sleep for six hours, for instance, allow a total of seven hours in bed. (This is a general guideline which may need to be adjusted for certain conditions, of course.) Ironically, reducing the time in bed does not reduce sleep time, but rather strengthens sleep efficiency, and your bed will be a stronger queue for sleep. Ideally, room temperature should also be slightly cool to allow the B.T. to naturally lower. Once time and temperature is adjusted, consider stress.

While we can't control our stressors, we can control how we respond to stress and negative emotions that significantly impact sleep. The stress hormones that are elevated during the day continue to be elevated as you sleep. The more intense the daytime stressor, the more difficult it is to sleep at night. Therefore, controlling your response in the day creates an environment for sounder sleep at night. Dr. Jacobs offers practical tools to calm thoughts and emotions in the Relaxation Response (RR) in his sleep program, *Say Goodnight to Insomnia*.

Perhaps for many, the challenge is in the emotional transition from the daytime to the nighttime. A smooth transition is achieved by the balance of the conscious and subconscious mind, (another polar balance) as Sondra Kornblatt, author of *Restful Insomnia,* explains.

She compares the conscious mind to the minivan driver trailing a to-do list, while the subconscious mind is the raft rider drifting along without a helm. She shares many strategies to harmonize the body and the *dual mind* driver/drifter. The following playful analogy of the battle of the minds may help you prepare for restful sleep, or at least, restful insomnia.

The conscious mind, *mini-van driver*, takes on the masculine *task-oriented* character, while the sub-conscious mind *raft rider* cultivates a feminine *feeling-oriented* quality. This does not reflect a gender statement, but rather, the dual gender balance in all of us, even as our dual gender hormones in the right proportion, create well-being.

While the night raft rider sits in the passenger seat in the day, she is not sleeping but, rather, is an intimate companion to the day driver. As they pass by a hitchhiker, a damsel in distress, the day driver *(hubby)* stops to give her a lift, but the night rider *(wifey)* warns, "I wouldn't do that!" Yet hubby's *Good Samaritan deed* overrides. After the hitchhiker is gone, so is his wallet! Now he's more upset because he didn't listen to his intuitive *better half*. As the evening approaches, it gets worse.

They drive up to a ferry where they are supposed to leave the minivan and enter the ferry. Wifey is the ferry's designated driver, gently gliding around islands and through canals, where they will visit *ferrylands* as they rest in a deep sleep. Yet hubby is so emotionally charged that he insists on still driving; and as you can imagine, it's quite a turbulent night.

Thus, to prepare for good sleep, we must allow for the transition of the dual minds. As we lie down, our *driving, thinking* side needs to visualize that we are now at the ferry, turn off the van, and get into the ferry, where the *feeling, riding* side can take us into a wonderland of rejuvenation. This is when you actually start to *feel* your feelings, both emotional and physical, and when your aching back groans. In *Restful Insomnia*, there are many strategies to help you *switch drivers* and retrieve feelings that are often suppressed in our body.

Quality sleep is one of the cornerstones for optimal health, yet so many of us are challenged in this area. Therefore, our wellness plan begins with developing habits that synchronize us with the natural circadian rhythm of the earth along with the use of gentle herbs and supplements to enhance sleep. Since many vitamins, minerals, and herbs work in concert together, there are blends that boost a synergistic effect, such as herbal teas and supplements like Advanced Sleep Formula by Advanced Bionutritionals. These are but a few possibilities, and the journey to sound sleep is different for each person. With natural remedies, hopefully you find that your journey is not a safari, at least until after you have fallen asleep.

Now that we have traveled the physical night journey, the following recommendations and readings can help make sleep an invigorating, positive experience, enhancing our appearance, mood, concentration, memory, immunity, and even libido!

Health Coach Recommendations

- Sleeping earlier rather than waking later will result in deeper, longer sleep. Increase energy by harmonizing your natural circadian rhythm with the sun's cycles of rising and setting. Wake up close to the same time every day.
- Avoid stimulants such as caffeine, sugar, (and for some, dairy) in the second half of the day.
- Avoid mental stimulations, such as viewing electronic devices before sleeping.
- Refrain from eating a few hours before sleeping, or snack lightly. The digestive system is also getting ready to sleep and doesn't digest food well in the night.
- Exercise daily to oxygenate the blood and cells, promoting deeper sleep.
- Drink water in the morning rather than before bedtime. Drinking a full glass of water (about 16 oz.) before any other drink or food in the morning flushes out the residue from

the night cleansing and increases energy throughout the day, while decreasing unhealthy cravings.

- Consider a hormonal checkup with a natural hormone doctor. Since hormones control our sleep quality, weight, energy, and affect all bodily systems, this could be your best health insurance and investment. (Anti-aging and regenerative medicine: A4M.com.)

Recommended Readings

Say Good Night to Insomnia by Gregg D. Jacobs
Restful Insomnia by Sondra Kornblatt

Spiritual Reflection of Light through Darkness

As plants sprout from the dark soil, and as an embryo grows encased in darkness, so life emanates from darkness. Emotional and spiritual *growth spurts* often occur during our dark times. Our greatest challenges of crisis, losses, and tragedies propel us into new breakthroughs, opportunities, relationships, and fresh perspectives. Losing a job may lead to an unbelievable enterprise, as it did for the founders of Home Depot; an unbearable tragedy might become a life-saving organization, such as the *Amber Alert*; or *getting dumped* may bring the love of your life! Our *Master Recycler* refurbishes the darkness into light as we cast our care on Him.

We see this powerful paradox played out in the lives of our *Genesis fathers and mothers, such as*: Noah, Abraham and Sarah, Isaac and Rebecca, Jacob and Rachel, and Joseph and his brothers. Their transformations might help us capture our own *big picture,* developed in our own *dark rooms.*

As I watch these breathtaking Genesis stories roll across the big screen of real life, I am amazed and humbled, for there too, is portrayed the grand story of humanity, winding through the tunnel of darkness into the light. Two remarkable themes interwoven in Genesis bring this journey full circle: the *progression* of the seed and *deception* of the seed. We too, as partakers of the promised seed, are challenged in this thread of deception, beginning with the first *deceiver* and the *deceived.*

Of course, it all begins with Eve deceived by the serpent, and Adam, yes, standing by his woman, coerced along, even as he justifies it; and their son, Cain, seemingly trying to deceive God with *leftovers* or a halfhearted sacrifice.

Then there's Noah, a man of marathon faith, whose human side leaves the door wide open to an unspeakable seduction.

What about Abraham (Abram), the father of our faith? Yes, he too, deceived not once, but twice, saying that Sarah (Sarai) was his sister, almost causing a great calamity. And Sarai too, deceived her husband as she was trying to help God cultivate the promised seed.

Ironically, Isaac displayed similar deceptive issues as his father, by the misrepresentation of his marital relationship; and by the end of his life, was deceived by his own son and wife, resulting in a generational turmoil for Esau, forfeiting his birthright.

Jacob, who was once the deceiver, is himself deceived when Laban gives him Leah instead of Rachel, and again, at the end of his second term of servitude, is tricked by his father-in-law to be, who once embraced him saying, "You are my own flesh and blood." Jacob, however, ultimately deceives his deceiver, leaving with the loot: both brides, many children, and a healthy productive prime flock. Rachel, too, turns out to be quite a match for her trickster hubby.

The Saga continues with Joseph's brothers who bring heart wrenching deceit to their own father by providing false evidence of his beloved son's death and then manipulating Joseph, too. Joseph is then falsely accused when he refuses to submit to the crafty Potiphar's wife. Joseph then deceives his brothers until he reveals himself.

Finally, Tamar's treachery leads to an irreversible predicament with Judah.

Now consider, as we are the *progression* of the seed, the prophesied countless *sand* and *stars.* How does this *deception* play out in our own lives?

We have probably all been, at some point, the *deceiver* or the *deceived* (or both), often deceiving ourselves. It is this subtle form of deception, which prevents us from entering into the Promised Land and compromising our health and happiness. Self-deception is elusive because we cannot separate *us* from ourselves for a reality check; only by prayer can we discern the indiscernible.

For instance, through our own self-limiting beliefs (usually played repeatedly in our internal dialogue) we might barter our *spiritual birth rights* of peace, prosperity and perfect health. Do we see our true image – expressing the love and powerful presence of God? Or are we deceived by ourselves, only seeing "our" potential, rather than The Lord's potential? Do we bring catastrophe by our own impatience of waiting for *the promised seed* to blossom in our own lives?

Just as Joseph prevailed through his series of events, so the Lord brings us full circle, through our series of misfortunate events, revealing His divine dream for our lives.

As Jonah's dark excursion led him through the belly of the whale, so our full journey with Christ takes us full circle through our own experiences by His death, burial, and resurrection, to become as *He is.* We are re-created in Christ as His amazing masterpiece, sculpted by His glorious *light,* where deception cannot hide. Likewise, our spiritual wellness blossoms as we unveil our true identity of the Lord's image in us; we become the stunning replica of Christ that emanates light wherever we go. And as we fully trust Him, He recycles our ashes into beauty, and our darkness into light. That's His specialty!

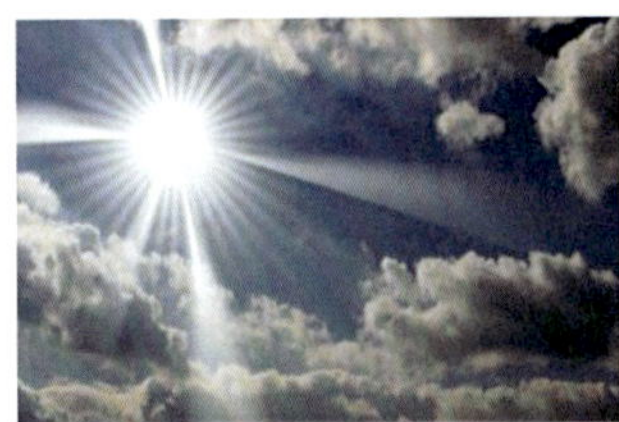

CHAPTER 2

The Healing Power of Light

Plants and Animals

"And God said, "Let there be light…" (Genesis 1:3)

It was one of those torrid lightning storms. Mother Nature rudely cut off the lights! Then she displayed her own fiery strobe light show of flashing lightning veins darting through the night fog, across the misty clouds, with full surround sound of shattering, crackling thunder.

Afterwards, my roommate walked past broken, dangling branches, surveying what was left of his vegetable garden. He stood astounded. The garden had not only survived but *thrived* brighter and greener than before, and even sprouted *several inches taller* immediately after the storm!

Certainly, plants flourish with fresh abundant rainfall and cool temperatures, but something significant accelerated this much growth, within just a few hours.

Lightning is a natural fertilizer, converting nitrogen in the air into a usable form, boosting instant plant development. The intense heat from electrical charges causes nitrogen to bond with oxygen, producing chlorophyll production by supercharged nitrogen doses.

As chlorophyll absorbs light energy, it triggers photosynthesis, producing food from natural sunlight. Plants are *instinctively* drawn to sunlight; just watch them bow, bend, crawl, or climb to touch the sunrays. If light energy accelerates plant development so exceedingly, imagine what it might do for us.

After the storm, my other roommate, *Oreo*, of the four legged kind, slithered out from under my bed where this big, bold *lion hid* during the thunder storm. When sunlight reappears, he once again sunbathes outside or in front of a window. So strong is his innate need for sunlight that he will bend into the formation of any sliver of light, like his feline friend, *Scamper*, squelching into a narrow ray of light.

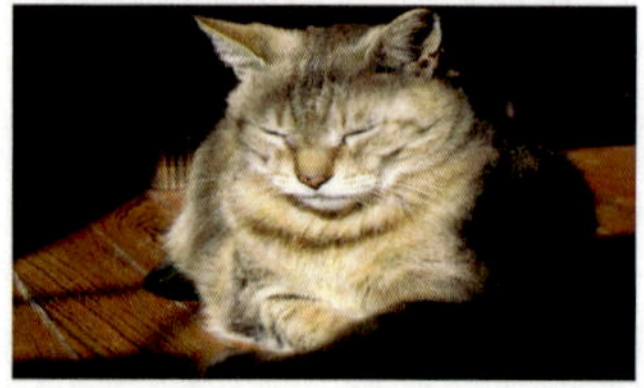

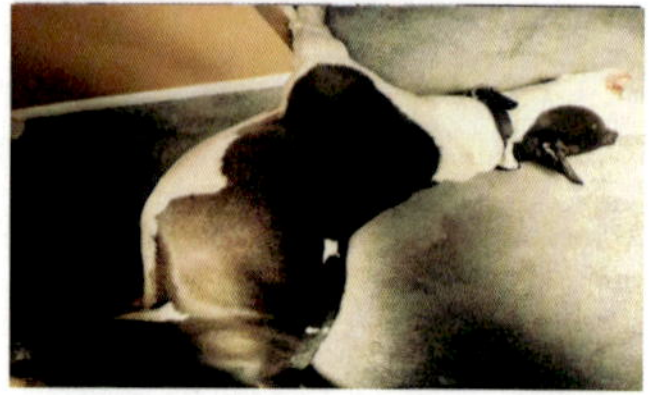

Perhaps our first step towards wellness is realizing that we, too, are mammals. Sunlight is crucial to our strong immunity and elevated physical and emotional well-being. Oreo proves his link to humanity when he climbs in bed, digs back the sheets, places his head on the pillow, and then snuggles under the covers. (Try convincing *him* that he's *not human.)*

Other animals also respond remarkably to UV light. In a 1925 study, hens were shown to produce ***four times*** as many eggs when exposed to a UV lamp. In later research, more benefits were discovered, such as increased hatching, thicker shells resulting in less breakage and more protection from infection, increased growth of chicks, earlier feathering, reduced disease, smaller feed required, and plumper, richer color.

In contrast, animals malnourished of sunlight (***mal-illumination***) display emotional imbalance that often results in violent and addictive behavior. For instance, rats in cages exposed to sunlight will be calm and manageable, but in continued light deficiency, will begin to attack the young. In another 1971 study, rats under stress preferred drinking water to alcohol, but when left in continuous darkness over the weekend, they went on alcoholic binges. (Now that's a new twist on "one drunk rat!")

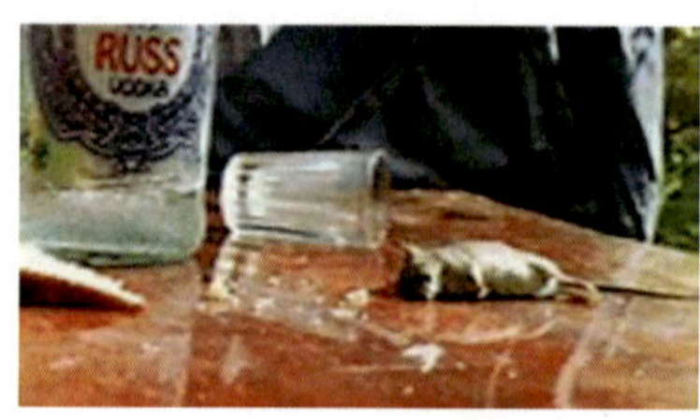

Starting to feel the human link? Our own biology, programmed for light, like plants and animals, might inspire us to respond to our own mammal instinctive need for sunlight.

We now turn to amazing *human* stories (as *illuminated* in "Into The Light" by William Campbell Douglass II, MD), from doctors who harnessed the power of penetrating sunlight and pioneered the health benefits of sunlight therapy, back in the *light ages* of the last century.

Humankind

Prior to modern sanitization practices, ultraviolet light has long been used as an effective sterilization method in commercial and medical uses. Some washing machines had a built-in ultraviolet light since it was well known that UV had an anti-bacterial effect. Toilet seats were also sanitized by sunlight. This common knowledge gave birth to the most profound anti-bacterial effect of light in medical practice. These exhilarating stories of breakthrough life-saving light therapies began back in the day of candlelight and the incandescent light.

In the dawning of the 20th century, doctors and researchers were making *light-year* discoveries of the amazing healing power of light in a process known as "photoluminescence." This long technical term is simply the combination of "photo" (*light)*, and "luminescence" (*emission of light)*. Thus, light was emitted both *externally* and *internally*, for a cornucopia of therapeutic applications. This revolutionary method was a safe, effective treatment.

External light therapy *came to light* by a Danish medical researcher, Niels Finsen, the Father of ultraviolet radiation therapy, back in the 1880s. He began treating "incurable" infectious skin disease with ultraviolet (UV) light treatments. The results were astonishing. More than 2,000 patients were treated for various skin diseases, with a 98% success rate, by exposing affected skin to sunlight.

Finsen's *enlightenment* led to an amazing discovery. He wondered if this healing was due to sunlight directly exposed to the affected skin, or if it was the effect of light internally, on the immune system. He treated some patients with sunlight funneled into the affected area alone, and others with sunlight on the whole body. The conclusion was astounding; the results were the same. The infection was not altered by the direct light itself, but rather, by light stimulating the *internal* immune process.

Finsen was awarded the Nobel Prize in physiology and medicine in 1903 for his photochemotherapeutic work. This was given "in recognition of his contribution to the treatment of diseases, especially lupus vulgaris (tuberculosis – like skin disease), with concentrated light radiation, whereby he has opened a new avenue for medical science." In 1904, Queen Alexandra visited his clinic, giving further credibility to his therapy, with many successors exploring the curative effects on many diseases.

Following Finsen's medical breakthrough, Dr. Auguste Rollier founded a sun clinic in the Swiss Alps, above the cloud layer, called *Le Chalet*. He developed a healing art by merging the therapeutic use of sunlight, a balanced diet, exercise, fresh air, and rest. Once again, this sun therapy program led to cures for "incurable" diseases in this pre-antibiotic time.

The sun-oriented rooms had large glass windows with a bed in an adjoining balcony. Patients were exposed to a few hours of morning or late afternoon sun in the summer and increased exposure in the winter. The results were incredible. Patients with spinal tuberculosis completely recovered, becoming healthy, functional, and with straightened backs. Many recovered from non-healing wounds such as abscesses, bone infections, and rickets. By 1940, Dr. Rollier opened over 30 sun clinics where he was able to treat over 1,000 people a day.

In these sun clinics, there was no incidence of skin cancer because patients were allowed to gradually acclimatize to the sun without getting sunburned. Sun exposure was early morning and late afternoon to prevent sunburn. (It's the overexposure to the sun, when sunburn occurs, that increases the risk of common skin cancer and causes premature aging of the skin, including wrinkles and dark spots.) Sunlight therapy was moderate and gradual.

While the results of these sunbathing clinics were most amazing, however, the *internal* method of *irradiating the blood*, known as "hemo-irradiation," was most astonishing, causing a direct, *laser* effect on the blood.

A small amount of blood (about 1/25th) was extracted, and an anti-coagulant was added to prevent clotting. It was then *irradiated* with UV light in a closed, air-tight circuit. The blood was immediately returned into the same vein from which it was drawn, thereby circulating the beneficial light energy into the entire bloodstream. This process neutralized toxins, empowering the normal immune system to finish destroying foreign organisms. Furthermore, it created a balancing act, regulating and normalizing the whole bodily system.

When blood cells were stimulated by ultraviolet light, all invaders were destroyed: viral, fungal, or bacterial, no matter how deeply hidden in the body! Patients rebounded rapidly from an array of diseases and near death illnesses. All toxins were quickly deactivated by this process. Patients usually recovered from even deadly poisons, such as snake or scorpion venom, or bacterial, such as strep and botulin, within just 24 to 72 hours! Serious conditions were treated, even tumors responded remarkably.

In 1928, Mr. Emmett K. Knott irradiated the blood of his first human subject, a patient with a fatal case of sepsis (bloodstream infection), after an abortion. The attending physicians declared this case hopeless, but after irradiation, she began a rapid recovery and later bore a normal child. Mr. Knott worked with Dr. Virgil K. Hancock and developed this therapy for many varieties of infections. Dr. Hancock used blood-irradiation to treat a patient of bloodstream infection with a temperature rising to 108.4 F, bone marrow infection, and bronchial pneumonia (considered a hopeless case, especially in the 1930s). This patient made a full recovery, as did many other patients, in moribund condition.

This method of exposing blood to light used UV rays to irradiate the bloodstream, thereby combatting all bloodstream infections. Doctors and researchers were successfully developing this amazing medical art and discovering further biological benefits. Dr. Hancock listed many surprising effects, such as deactivating of toxins and viruses, destroying bacteria growth, increasing oxygen in the blood and cells, and activating steroids and vitamin D. Blood irradiations frequently increased red blood cells as high as 1.2 million over night, while white cells balanced to normal levels.

The brilliant *light baton* was passed on to more successors. In the 1930s, Dr. George Miley demonstrated the curative impact of increased oxygen absorption in the blood after ultraviolet exposure. This was a monumental discovery because oxygen absorption greatly increases energy, promoting healing. Dr. Miley recorded phenomenal results in 151 cases of acute infections: a 100% recovery of those treated early, 98% recovery in moderately advanced cases, and 42% in moribund cases. One patient dying of botulinum, unable to swallow or see, fully revived within days. Many with viral pneumonia had completely cleared cough and lungs within a few days. By 1942, 6,520 patients had been treated with an exceedingly high success rate and complete absence of any harmful effects in his detailed clinical observations of hundreds of patients he treated over the years in Pennsylvania hospitals. One can only marvel at the successful recoveries in this *pre-antibiotic era.*

According to Dr. Miley, "The toxins in the bloodstream… exposed to UV radiation (are) inactivated…and beneficial energy (is) stored up in the rayed blood temporarily, and if such blood can be returned to the bloodstream immediately…, it will throw off secondary irradiation which will stimulate and energize the patient."

Dr. Miley said that the groundbreaking contribution of Mr. Knott was "… one of the greatest contributions to medicine ever made by a citizen of the United States. There is as yet no other therapy capable of producing the same results." Let the medical records prove that the same is true today.

These are only a few of the thousands who utilized this gift of light. It's mind-boggling to imagine how blood can be exposed to UV for only a few seconds and then returned to internally irradiate the whole bloodstream, reaping the full potential of light. Yet to me, it's even more incomprehensible that such a simple, effective, responsive, yet *inexpensive* treatment was laid to rest. "*Inexpensive,*" perhaps that *is* the key word.

PHOTOLUME PROCEDURE

This describes procedure after set-up and connection of dual male luer lock, proximal IV tubing, quartz cuvette, distal IV tubing, 3-way stopcock/5cc syringe/60cc syringe.

1. Heparin Preparation
   a. 3 cc's of 10,000/per cc of heparin into 30 cc of sterile saline.
   b. 5 cc's of above mix in 5 cc syringe
2. Heparinizing System
   a. Draw 5 cc's of mixture through stopcock into 50 cc syringe and coat walls
   b. Push this solution through closed tubing system until reaching end.
   c. Collect 3 cc's of heparin mixture and attach to stopcock.
3. Treatment
   a. Turn on instrument
   b. Attach the connector set to the winged infusion in patient's arm
   c. Draw blood into the 60 cc syringe through the light and return back into patient
   d. After 1st cycle TURN OFF LIGHT
   e. Inject into the 60 cc syringe the 3 cc's of Heparin attached to stopcock (If 3 cycles to be done repeat Step II-c).
   f. Draw Heparin in. DO NOT PUSH INTO PATIENT:
   g. Repeat Step II-C, leaving Heparin solution (approximately 3cc) in 60 CC syringe.
   h. TURN LIGHT BACK ON!
   i. Pull patient's blood through light into 60-cc syringe then return patient's blood.

   This completes 2nd cycle
4. Completion of Procedure
   a. Detach patient-end of connector set and reattach IV to keep vein open

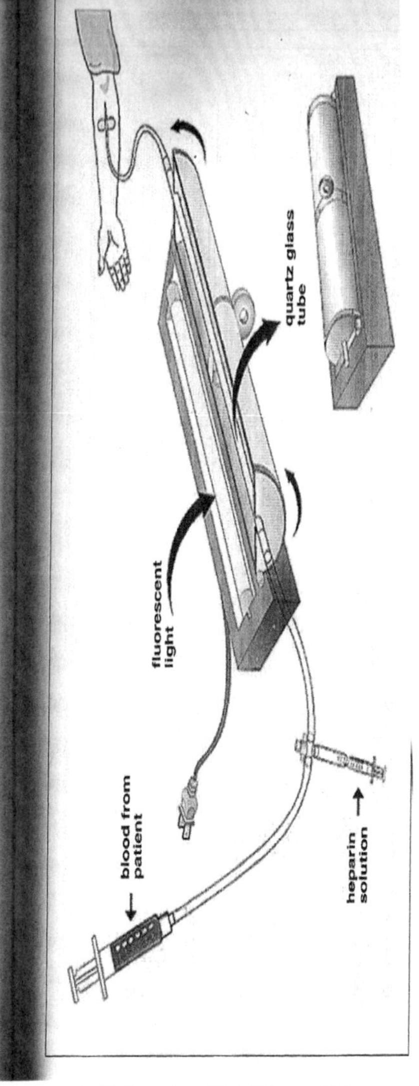

"Into The Light" by William Campbell Douglass II, MD, pg. 254

Back to the Future

If we only knew *now* what we knew *then*, perhaps we could have saved the life of Jim Henson, the creator of the Muppets, who died of streptococcal toxemia in 1990. Photoluminescent therapy might have immediately neutralized such toxins, but it *was not used.*

Now, here's the million dollar question (literally, the million dollar question). If this technique is so effective and safe, why isn't it a common practice in today's medicine?

The tremendous progress of photoluminescence, (*with no side effects)*, faded away when antibiotics, such as penicillin, came on the scene. Why on earth would progressive medicine abandon this incredible breakthrough, proven to cure otherwise *incurable* diseases, even when antibiotics don't work?

Of course, antibiotics have great beneficial value today and have also saved countless lives, but why not fight the war on disease with all of our ammunition? Why abandon this extremely successful, yet simple, lifesaving method?

For instance, photo (light) chemotherapy targets only the *abnormal cells*, which, when subjected to the light, destroys them. Photo-sensitive dyes are injected and the irradiated blood tags *only the diseased cells*. The photo activated antibody specifically illuminates the *enemy* and removes it from the bloodstream while preserving the healthy cells, leaving them unaffected. Cancer cells tend to absorb more photosensitive chemicals than normal cells, and therefore, certain light frequencies completely kill the cancer. Therefore, there is a much greater chance of continued remission with light therapy. Initially, the light-activated drug is absorbed by all cells, but cancer cells retain the drug longer. In two days, it remains only in the tumor cells. Laser light then allows the drug to release a toxic form of oxygen, destroying only the cancer cells. Since this process selectively destroys only cancer cells, the patient has a strong immunity army for recovery, while averting the terrible side effects of chemotherapy.

Globally we are spearheading great advancements as light therapy warriors conquer or at least make vast improvements in warring the *Goliaths* of heart disease, diabetes, mental imbalances, cancer, and even AIDS!

Many hospitals in Russia have used light therapy for hypertension with as much as a 30% lowering of high blood pressure and decrease in chest pain and headaches. Blood irradiation resulted in a 90% lower rate of heart attacks in patients with severe angina pectoris, compared to only 30% of those not receiving light therapy. Arrhythmia (irregular heart beat) was also treated with an 81% success rate in contrast to 33% without light therapy. Intensive UV therapy was so effective that many patients avoided surgical heart valve repair. What a remarkable accomplishment! As for those who needed surgery, Russian doctors who used intra-aortal light therapy (introducing light into the aorta) saw many benefits with greatly accelerated recovery and reduced mortality rate.

UV blood irradiation reduced blockage of arteries in the legs, a common problem for diabetic and other conditions, and stabilized blood sugar. Patients reported significant pain relief, increased circulation, better sleep, and better appetite. In this delicate procedure, laser light is inserted directly into a vein or artery. An intravenous drip is applied in the large vein in the arm. Then a hair-like fiber optic thread is connected whereby the light travels down the thread and radiates the blood.

Additionally, light therapy has been a lifesaver for many AIDS patients. Many hospitals and clinics in Africa and abroad use Photo-Oxidation (photoluminescence combined with photo-oxidation drugs) to allow AIDS patients to live with greater strength and stability. One of the first benefits is rejuvenating the liver, which then revitalizes the whole bodily system. Thus, they experience not only greater longevity, but also a healthier quality of life.

UV irradiation also helps the body rid itself of uric acid, a considerable treatment for gout (an arthritic condition of uric acid deposit in the joints). Patients suffering from rheumatoid arthritis reported extraordinary improvement within a few hours of treatment, and some arthritis cleared completely.

The marvelous effect of light therapy on the autonomic nervous system has a myriad of benefits on the body's response system, especially on the digestive and respiratory. For instance, paralysis of the bowels is rapidly relieved by UV blood irradiation as the autonomic nervous system which controls the gastrointestinal tract returns to normal function. Similarly, asthma dramatically responds as it relaxes, smoothing the bronchial muscles.

Finally, UV therapy has been used to stabilize many mental imbalances or disorders. Light is used as an anti-depressant for S.A.D (seasonal affective disorder). There's also been proven results in other conditions such as hyperactivity.

Our *Solar Systems*

We have seen the almost magical effect of UV light on our blood both in times past and in other countries. Another great pioneer in the field of photobiology is Dr. John Ott. In the 1980s, he demonstrated how the full-spectrum of light is absolutely essential for good health in all life forms. Dr. Ott conducted a study on how light impacts the behavior of children. In a grade school in Sarasota, Florida, he arranged full spectrum florescent lights in one classroom and non-full spectrum lights in the other classroom. Children who were exposed to full spectrum light exhibited a marked decrease in hyperactivity with a calming effect, even in those with a "confirmed learning disability." Furthermore, those under full spectrum light had other health benefits, such as decreased cavities.

Dr. Ott also reminded medical associates of the value of light therapy for infants. Since the 1950s, it's been recommended to treat jaundice in newborn babies with photo therapy using *blue light* which enables the babies' systems to break down the excess bilirubin serum in the blood (more about color lights in chapter 3).

Furthermore, Dr. Ott highly recommended using full-spectrum lights (which resemble natural daylight) in facilities such as hospitals, daycares, schools, doctors' offices, and nursing homes where sanitization is crucial. According to a study by Duke University, properly installed and maintained full spectrum lights *eliminates 75 -95% of viable bacteria in the air*, with a drastic drop in the infection rate! This method disinfects the air quite efficiently because normal air currents cause bacteria to rise and fall from the floor about once per minute. As bacteria are carried into the ultraviolet rays near the ceiling, they are destroyed or weakened. This highly proficient method of disinfecting the air is equivalent to changing the room air about once every minute!

Ott believes that there is a strong link between chronic disease and lack of sunlight. Another primary entrance of light is through our eyes into our chief photoreceptor, the pineal gland, which protects us from light deficiency. Therefore, Dr. Ott warns not to obstruct this natural process by wearing UV blocking sunglasses. The pineal gland is also the main communication center for hormone production, regulating all of our bodily systems. Estrogen, an essential hormone for conception, sharply peaks with UV absorption, which is filtered out by most sunglasses. Dr. Ott advised six patients who were unable to conceive to throw away their tinted sunglasses, and indeed, they all conceived! The same concept may well hold true for the male hormone. Sunlight and adequate hormone production also shield us from disease.

Dr. Ott noted the comment of Dr. Albert Schweitzer in Africa, who said that after the sunglass craze, there was a dramatic increase of cancer. Light deficiency is even more profound in dark skin, which does not absorb UV light as well as light skin. Therefore, shielding UV light through the eyes has an even more dramatic effect, especially for those of dark skin.

Dr. Ott added, "My studies have indicated that light is a nutrient, similar to all other nutrients we take in through food, and that we need full spectrum range of natural daylight. This fact has long been proven by science." In 1967, three Russian scientists concluded, "If human skin is not exposed to solar radiation (direct or scattered light) for long periods of time, disturbances will occur in the physiological equilibrium of the human system. The result will be functional disorders of the nervous system and a vitamin D deficiency, a weakening of the body's defenses, and an aggravation of chronic diseases."

Dr. Ott compares some of the skin receptors with solar cells used in our satellites to energize them from the sun. He sees the Langerhans cells of the skin as a computer-like, semiconductor chip that energize us directly from the sun, just like plants, only in a different way. The layers of skin are like the layers of elements used to make transistors, a complex electro photo-magnetic receiving system, and are our biological solar energy cells. Yes, we truly are solar powered! How amazingly we have been created!

10 Sunshine Benefits

Natural sunshine may well be one of the best health insurance policies and totally free! We need to protect ourselves from *lack of sun*, but moderately, avoiding even slight sunburn. Feel the amazing sunshine benefits:

1. **Increases Energy:** Sunlight accelerates energy production, and our energy level parallels our overall health, even slowing the rate of aging. This occurs on a deeper level and on broader range than we may immediately feel.

2. **Maintains Healthy Weight:** Sunlight stimulates the metabolic rate in both people and animals, which controls weight management, appetite, and digestive hormones.

3. **Boosts Immunity:** Notice how flu symptoms and related sickness are triggered primarily in the later winter months when we haven't had much sun exposure for a few months. In a 1979 study by *The British Journal of Medicine,* the vitamin D levels of seniors was tracked for sixteen months. In November, levels dropped by an average of *19%*, but by February, it was an alarming *65%*. These extremely low levels are associated with the development of Osteoporosis and other disease.

4. **Promotes Calcium in Bones and Teeth:** Vitamin D production is stimulated by sunlight and promotes calcium absorption into the bones and teeth. When calcium is not properly absorbed, deposits pool in other areas such as joints, causing pain and stiffness, and in arteries, causing potentially fatal plaque accumulation, which can lead to heart issues. It is crucial that calcium is channeled properly with adequate blood levels of Vitamin D3.
5. **Controls Cancer:** Vitamin D is crucial in harnessing the immune system to control cancer. Low levels are especially associated with breast and prostate cancer.
6. **Heals Psoriasis:** Sunlight exposure is a healing balm for psoriasis. In a four week sunbathing therapy study, 84% of participants experienced significant clearance of psoriasis.
7. **Elevates Mood:** Sunshine is a natural anti-depressant that actually increases serotonin, our mood-lifting chemical, which our brains produce more of on sunny days.
8. **Improves Alzheimer's:** Full-spectrum daylight improves some aspects of Alzheimer's disease, such as reducing agitation and nighttime activity, including insomnia.
9. **Enhances Quality of Sleep:** Sunlight in the day helps ensure adequate melatonin in the night (the hormone that helps you sleep). Low levels of melatonin are associated with poor sleep quality, especially in older adults.
10. **When possible,** let us bask outdoors in the full spectrum of the sun as do our fellow canine and feline friends. Like an orchid, let us bow, bend, crawl, or climb over obstacles of time and space and stretch to catch the sunrays. We have seen how light truly enlightens our whole life and health, and here are some ways we can soak up the rays.

Modern Use of Light Therapies

Over the years, light therapy has been increasingly used in combination with surgery, radiation, and many other traditional treatments. I have personally used light as an antibiotic with IV antibiotics, boosting an impressive recovery.

Crystal Light Therapy is another form of medicinal lights gaining popularity with versatile applications such as supporting chemotherapy and infectious disease treatment. This unique medicinal art combines crystals, guided meditation, sound and essential oils with therapeutic massage. Color light is infused into the seven major chakras of the auric and physical body, while resting comfortably under several crystal cannons, or a single colored light, as seen below. Each crystal aligns with the corresponding chakra color, and are set on a special vibrational frequency to create balance of mind, body, and soul, thereby removing energy blocks and opening the natural healing channels. Various conditions determine precise light distances. Crystal Light Therapists can be found online, and we'll explore the medicinal colors in chapter 3.

As we come to understand the full spectrum values of this therapy, not as a standalone cure-all approach, but as a powerful complementary modality especially when paired with the array of other healing arts, in both conventional and alternative therapies. This is only a brief overview of the amazing medical science of light therapy today.

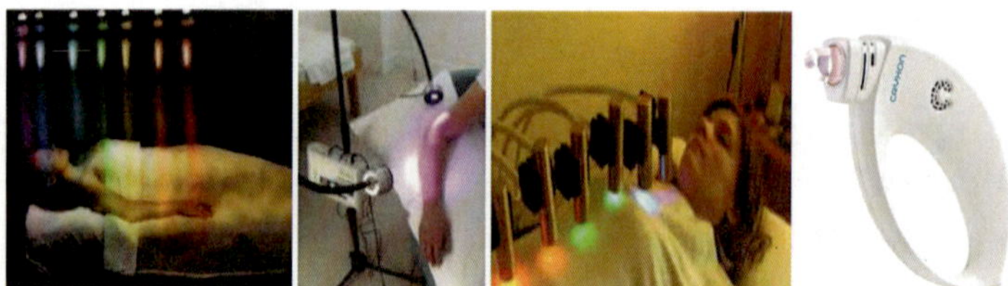

Crystals and gemstones are dynamic healing tools because of their piezoelectric effect. Crystals and gemstones respond to the electricity that is coursing through our body, transforming energy by the constant electrical vibrations of the stones which help to harmonize, balance, and stimulate these energies.

The revolutionary crystal lamp, Cryxon (pictured on far right) is a complex, digitally controlled device combining the beneficial effects of the different types of healing crystals, special lights and colors.

Natural sunlight, being full spectrum light, is certainly an optimal light source too. Sunlight pouring through multicolored stained glass windows or doors for example helps to balance all seven chakras simultaneously with light. So the next time you are sitting under a stained glass window at church, consider it a double blessing.

Health Coach Recommendation

- Plan outdoor fun, like walking, playing, or lounging, for 15 minutes of daily sun.
- Take indoor activities outdoors, such as eating, reading, and using phone and laptop.
- Create an outdoor mini office or sun chair to engage in play, work, reading, and writing, eating, meditating, praying, or just resting, at or near your home.
- Cover your face when sun bathing. Facial skin is thin and already gets excess sun.
- Minimize sun lotion to times of excess sun exposure, since it blocks the sun benefits.
- Consider light therapy treatment for any disease or condition, especially if your current therapy is not working. (Contact trained specialist for help with this.)

Recommended Reading

Into the Light by William Campbell Douglass II, MD

Spiritual Reflection of Light

As we have seen, light has supernatural healing power. Now see the physical properties of light glittering in the *reflecting pool* of spiritual light.

God is light; in him there is no darkness at all. (I John 1:5)

God is light; the piercing light that penetrates our whole being, infiltrates every cell, and initiates healing throughout all of our bodily systems. No disease can hide! No sickness can exist in the presence of the glorious light, not even the *Goliaths*, as even the *incurable* is cured. No disease is permanent; only the Word of God prevails forever, dispelling darkness.

God is *The Light* shining through the sacred blood line since the beginning, conquering the impenetrable walls of darkness, to preserve His seed, that one day there would be *children of light*.

This Light is a fire that purifies seven times (completely complete). It burns the chaff of shame, anger, and doubt. *This light* searches and purges the deep issues hidden in the shadows of the heart and clothes us with the *righteous robe of light*.

His Light shines in many forms and in many ways. Sometimes its rays touch our lives as words of hope, acts of compassion, a gentle touch, or prayer and praise that radiates through every circumstance, even when all is dark. Light accelerates healing, stimulates growth, and promotes health in all of life.

Your word is a lamp to my feet and a light to my path. (Psalm 119:105 NASB)

When we bask in *The Light*, we become *solar powered*. His thoughts become our thoughts. We walk *in the light* by faith, in the *full spectrum* of His word, and receive both physical and spiritual healing.

We absorb His *enlightening* wisdom that discerns the indiscernible, separating thoughts from intents, even bone from marrow. We are infused with joy, compassion, and all of the fruit of the spirit ripens in full blossom on a vine in the fullness of *Sonshine*.

In concluding the benefits of full spectrum light, we'll now look into the sky at the specific healing attributes in the colors of the rainbow. Each color emits a healing balm to the human body. In the next chapter, we'll explore color light therapy by two admirable *lights in this world,* Dr. Dinshan Ghadiali (1873 – 1966), affectionately known as the reviver of color light therapy and inventor of the Spectro-Chrome technology; and Dr. Kate W. Baldwin (1855-1935), an amazing, renowned surgeon who colored *outside of the lines,* healing many, while stirring up the powers that be. (Sound familiar?)

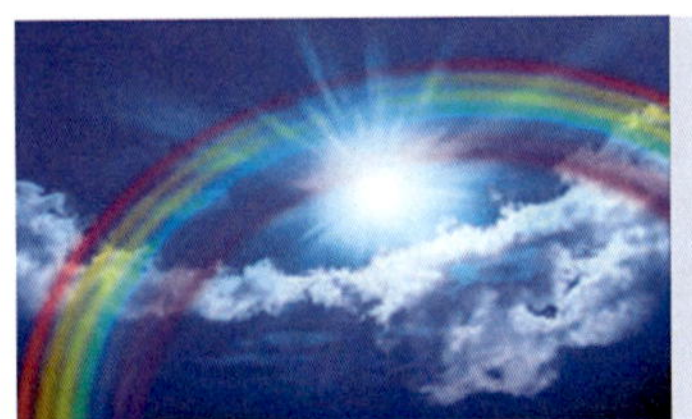

CHAPTER 3
The Healing Power of the Rainbow

I will put my rainbow in the clouds to be a sign of my promise to the earth. (Genesis 9:13 GWT)

In 1672, Sir Isaac Newton discovered the *color spectrum* as he was passing by the window of a drug store. He noticed that the light coming through a jar displayed a complete rainbow on the other side. He concluded that light is made up of various colors, and when combined, make white light. Through the ages, others began unraveling the light mystery.

In 1878, Dr. Edwin Dwight Babbitt presented the biological effects of the light spectrum in his book, *The Principles of Light and Color*. He said, "It is quite time that the wonder of light and color…should be made known many mysteries of nature and human life…"

Indeed, it was time! Yet, unfortunately, it was before its time, and *still is*! Pioneer, Dr. Denshah Ghadiali, was so far ahead of *his time* that most of the medical world is still (about 100 years later), vastly unaware of the amazing power of color. He was an incredible genius who demonstrated the relentless compassion of our Lord and reception of higher wisdom, while severely and unjustly penalized for his healing wonders.

About 1890, Dr. Ghadiali had a dramatic vision, leading to the revelation of the healing powers in the promise of the rainbow. He reached up, and touching the colors of the sky, began to develop the healing art of color science with a machine which he invented, the *Spectro-Chrome.*

Dr. Dinshah Ghadiali came to America from India to learn from his hero, Thomas Edison. He served in the New York Air Reserves as a Colonel, inventing many things. His genius led to his marvelous invention, the Spectro-Chrome. It was a rectangular machine with five specially tinted glass plate slides, projected by an incandescent bulb inside. The five glass plates could overlap to produce the specific color. According to Dinshah, light works to restore balance or "normalize" these energy centers. The healing of the physical body follows the restoration of the natural balance of the etheric body. If a certain element is lacking, it can be balanced by nourishing the etheric body with that attuned color. Likewise, when there's too much of a certain kind of energy, balance can be restored using the opposing (polar) color.

One day, he was called to the home of a woman fatally ill with mucous colitis and severe diarrhea, pain, and blood loss. After three days of conventional treatments, she cried out to the 24 year old Dr. Ghadiali, "Oh Denshah, save me!"

"Medically, she was beyond recovery, and I said to her, 'Call on the Almighty to save you, dear girl... I have no medicine of which I know can be of service to you, but…I shall endeavor to do my best otherwise.'"

This was his opportunity to test the chromo therapy he had learned from Dr. Babbitt. Since the woman was dying, Ghadiali reasoned, *I couldn't kill her if I failed.* He purchased a hurricane lamp and some colored pickle bottles to serve as color slides. Then, he applied to her abdomen the colors he surmised would be beneficial for this disease. By the next day, her bowel movements reduced, and in three days, she was out of bed.

"…Other experiences followed this one," said Ghadiali, "and my mind whirled with the intoxication of using higher forces of the physical plane for the alleviation of the ailments of humanity… the beauties of colors (are not) solely aesthetic… and decoration."

Ghadiali shares another story of a 19-year-old boy, almost moribund from advanced pulmonary tuberculosis. He placed the appropriate color frequency to his lungs, and within one and a half hours, the boy was sitting up in bed; and three hours later, he was eating dinner! The next morning, his father saw him up and eating breakfast with no apparent discomfort and said, "Colonel,

I now see why they call you a magician; I never thought I might see Paul alive again."

You would think that such a medical hero would be highly esteemed. Yet, this natural, powerful method became a threat to the pharmaceutical business. This incomprehensible wonder greatly threatened governmental powers.

"They showed up ten strong. A full-fledged FBI squad, and on…July 14, 1951, proceeded to lay out each and every one of the strange machines from Dr. Dinshah's clinic onto his lawn. With sledge hammers, they smashed each one to pieces as the old man, his patients, and neighbors watched. They wanted to deliver a message and did so. Dinshah was sentenced to three years in prison."

In fact, he was harassed during his entire career. In a 1930 trial, he represented himself, calling to the stand his physician-witness, Dr. Kate Baldwin. She was an extraordinary doctor serving as Senior Surgeon at Women's Hospital of Philadelphia for 23 years. She was a member of the American Academy of Ophthalmology and American College of Surgeons.

He asked Dr. Baldwin about a certain burn case of a little girl who was saved using color light therapy. Most of her body, and about four fifths of her torso, was so gruesomely burned that the skin was destroyed, including the fascia (covering) of the muscle, leaving only raw muscle exposed.

"From my…experience," said Dr. Baldwin, "it would be an absolutely hopeless and fatal case. I told myself that there was nothing in regular medicine or surgery that can make that child live…that we might as well see what the Spectro-Chrome will do. The child had absolutely nothing but color and diet. I used no surgery at all. I used paper dressing soaked with nut oil and color rays. We used turquoise principally to build the skin. We used other colors to help stimulate the separation of the sloughs off the body. New skin will not cover over dead tissue and we had to stimulate the separation using stimulating colors." (Another issue was that the child couldn't urinate for more than 48 hours. Scarlet light was applied over the kidneys, at a distance of about eighteen inches, for twenty minutes, and all other areas covered; two hours later, she voided.)

"Now, I was criticized for not skin grafting, but where could I get skin to graft? There was no place on the body to graft skin. Amazingly, Grace recovered by color therapy with perfectly moveable skin, not scar tissue - but skin!"

The highly respected Dr. Baldwin explained her perspective. "We will always need the undertaker...but anything that is in human possibility...can be done with Spectro-Chrome better than it can be done with anything else, and in many cases, it is the only thing that would put the patient in a condition to function."

When asked if she still used chromo therapy, she said, "I use practically nothing else...only in the matter of emergency would I use the old methods of treatment."

She added, "In many cases of cancer, if there has not been too much destruction of tissue, the Spectro-Chrome will cure it; it will build up the tissue. ... If there is a great deal of destruction of tissue, it will simply make them more comfortable so they can enjoy the rest of their lives to a certain extent, without doping them with opiates." She concluded, "...I would close my office tonight never to see another sick person, unless it was as emergency, if I had to go back to old style medicine and give up Spectro-Chrome."

Despite this stunning testimony, Dr. Ghadiali's institutions were burnt down, his inventions and publications destroyed, and he was sentenced and fined. Yet he was a very spiritual, intuitive, and serious scientist and a genius as an inventor and natural healer.

While the energetic and therapeutic potential of colors is

still greatly untapped in our world, many European countries, and especially Russia, utilize the healing colors. (Sadly, we tend to use color where it is *lucrative*, in advertising and electronics.)

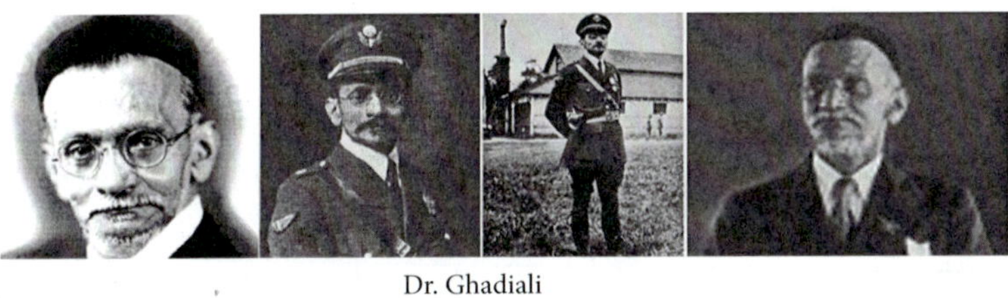

Dr. Ghadiali

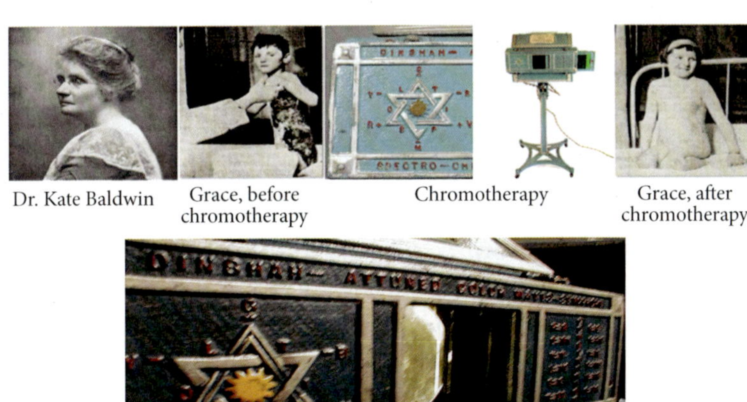

Dr. Kate Baldwin

Grace, before chromotherapy

Chromotherapy

Grace, after chromotherapy

What is Color Therapy and how does it work?

With these powerful testimonies, we must ask, *What is Chromo therapy*?

First, it is *not* magical, mystical, or new age; rather, it is a clinical, scientifically grounded science of the medicinal use of color.

The concept of treating illness by shining a specific color may sound like *something out there* in the star wars zone, but consider how we already use infrared and ultraviolet light. For example, infrared has a warming effect, allowing heat to penetrate deep into the tissue, and therefore has many applications.

Beyond the visible color is *vibratory energy*. Each color emanates certain electro-magnetic wave lengths, as sound does. For instance, red vibrates at 436 trillion times per second, while violet has 731 oscillations per second. Color doesn't penetrate the skin, but rather, the colors' wave lengths affect the electromagnetic *aura* surrounding the human body. Each of the seven colors corresponds with the seven chakras, subtle energy points located throughout the body. Each chakra is connected to a certain organ or part of the human body.

When color is absorbed through our outer shell, it *creates balance, relaxation, or stimulation,* depending on the color. This creative *energy* then restores the condition of our physical being. Our body responds to color, as do our minds, in various ways. It can soothe, stimulate, soften, strengthen, support, and balance our internal organs and bodily systems. Every color (and color combination) has a specific medicinal effect and an individual impression on each person. The auric body absorbs the color light wave length and then applies it as needed to the physical body.

The Spectro-Chrome enables 5 basic colors to create 12 total colors and the symmetry between them, as seen below. These colors have the power to heal or help almost any disease or condition, including cancer. Dinshah worked diligently for over 30 years documenting how various colors treat an array of illnesses. While he has written volumes, a condensed version of color combinations for healing almost 400 diseases and conditions can be found in his book, *Let there be Light*. You can also take a full tour of the original Spectro-Chrome on YouTube: the-return-of–the-spectro-chrome-the-most-suppressed-medical-technology.

His legacy still lives on in European countries, especially in England and Russia, and in South America and Asia where color therapy is commonplace in many medical facilities. He has left behind not only his inventions, but also precise color charts and applications. As Dr. Kate said, color therapy can cure about everything except broken bones and some diseases that are too advanced. Among the hundreds of conditions that color remedies can treat are addictions such as alcohol, drugs, cigarettes, and obesity. Color therapy is easy to learn, and anyone can order a modern light therapy kit on the internet or take online classes, all very inexpensively, to develop this wonderful healing art. I have provided these links at the end of this chapter and my personal testimonies. We will now finish as Dr. Kate Baldwin's expresses the wonders of the Spectro-Chrome:

"For centuries scientists have devoted untiring effort to discover means for the relief or cure of human ills and the restoration of the normal functions. Yet in neglected light and color, there is potency far beyond that of drugs and serums. Color is the simplest and most accurate therapeutic measure yet developed. I can produce more accurate results with colors than with any or all other methods combined – and with less strain on the patient."

History of Development of Color Light Therapy

The evolution of the science of color actually dates back to ancient Greece. Over time, this gem was unearthed and developed in medical practices. At the turn of the 19th century, this color system was developed by Johan Wolfgang van Goethe. He visually portrayed that light and darkness are the primary essences, and that color was created by their interaction. *Color appears, born as the offspring energy, where mother light, and father darkness meet.*

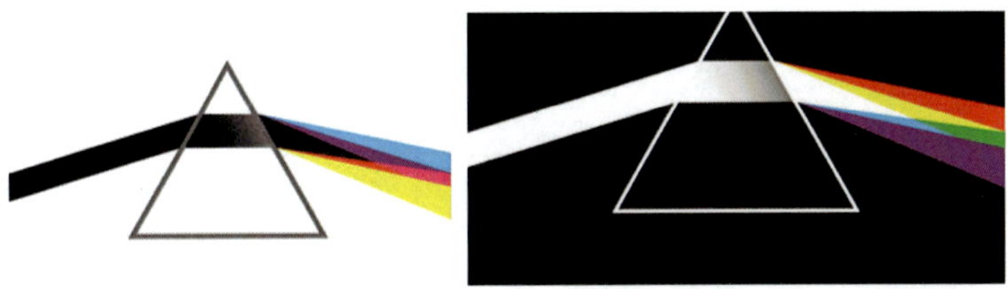

Darkness passing through light *Light passing through darkness*

Darkness seen through light creates soothing blues and dark deep colors (turquoise, blue, violet), in the upper half.

Light seen through darkness generates stimulating bright colors (red, yellow, orange). These rainbow colors surround green in the middle as the center color of balance and stability. Thus, green is the color of balance.

The following six point star (as pictured on the Spectro-Chrome) shows the precise medicinal properties of each color.

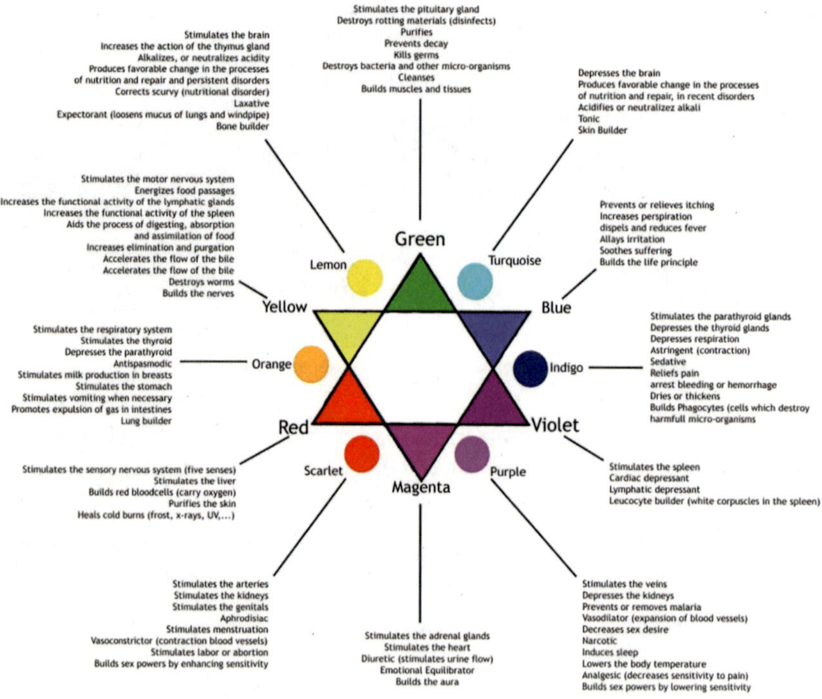

Notice the *polar colors* opposite each other in this ingenious color star. These opposing colors can even be used to *offset* each other. Cool soothing blues are on one side, and stimulating reds are on the other, with green, the balancing color, in the middle.

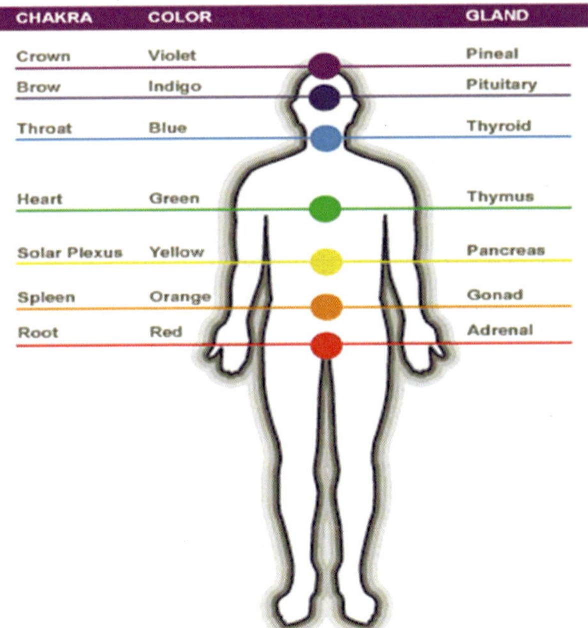

These *seven colors* of the rainbow correlate with the *seven chakras*. The numerical significance of seven is complete, (as in the seven days of creation). Thus, complete health is reflected in the seven colors matching the seven chakras, as follows. Warm colors (red, yellow, and orange) are stimulating and detoxifying, while the blues are relaxing and restoring.

RED Root Chakra, at the spinal base: (awakening and invigorating)

- Increases blood pressure, heart rate, pulse, breathing
- Activates the five senses by stimulating the sensory nervous system.
- Stimulates the liver and builds platelets and hemoglobin, purifying the blood.
- Expels toxins through the skin rapidly which may cause redness or itching until internal cleansing is complete.

- Use cautiously to prevent increasing fever and inflammation.

ORANGE Splenic Chakra, under the navel: (creative and rejuvenating)

- Heals digestive issues, relieves gas, cramps, spasms, and vomiting
- Improves lungs and is a respiratory stimulant, decongestant
- Improves thyroid and is a parathyroid depressant
- Stimulates mammary glands to increase milk production
- Improves bone health, stronger bones
- Stimulates tissue growth

YELLOW Solar Plexus Chakra, at Solar Plexus: (intellectual and communicator)

- Can raise or lower the mental and emotional state
- Energizes muscles by stimulating motor nervous system, repairs nerves
- Stimulates intestines, pancreas, digestive fluids
- Increases bowel movement, expels parasites
- Stimulates lymphatic system
- Depresses spleen

GREEN Heart Chakra, at center of heart: (balances emotions and bodily systems)

- Physical and emotional equilibrator
- Rebuilds muscle and tissue
- Stimulates and balances pituitary
- Regenerates and stabilizes the nervous system
- Cleanses and prevents decay

TURQUOISE Throat Chakra, at throat: (regenerating and relaxing)

- Heals inflammation in the body
- Rebuilds burned skin
- Relaxes the nervous system
- Reduces stress and anxiety

BLUE Third-Eye-Chakra, on the forehead: (intuition, mental projection)

- Relieves irritation and itching
- Mild sedative
- Reduces fever and inflammation
- Stimulates pineal gland

VIOLET The Crown-Chakra, on the top of the head: (activity and relaxation)

- Increases leucocytes, white blood cells
- Eases nervous system
- Depresses lymphatic glands and pancreas
- Builds spleen
- Decreases muscular activity, including the heart

Modern Use of Color Light Therapy

Today, anyone can easily learn how to effectively use this healing modality, thanks to the light therapy pioneers such as Dr. Dinshah, who studied and refined the benefits of Color Light therapy over his life of medical practice.

This gentle healing art has come a long way, since the early days when Dr. Dinshah first shined his flashlight through a colored pickle bottle. Later, through his invention of the Spectro-Chrome, he developed *gel* colored filters. These were cumbersome, requiring long *tonations* (duration of light sessions) and specifications, not to mention the tedious creation of accurate *schedules* (the order of lights used in each session.)

Light filters can be made with theatrical slides and the directions provided in "Let There Be Light," by Darius Dinshah, or an entire color light kit can be ordered for about $150 from Rose (don't you love how names often reflect professions) at: rose@coloredlighttherapy.com

The light therapy kit includes 10 numbered color glass filters producing 12 colors, a lamp, a 50-60watt bulb, and a filter holder built on the front of the lamp. The lamp has an attachment do it can be ~~to~~ set on top of a tripod, or it can set on most any heat-resistant surface. Also included are both the instructions for these filters, and Dinshah's book with light schedules of over 400 conditions and diseases.

Ideally, the lamp should be set up 3 to 5 feet from the patient, because it needs to be outside of the etheric body so that it can absorb, and process the energy within the physical body. This amazing phenomenon happens through the energy centers, the Chakras, which then direct the healing internally, into the physical body as needed. The exception to this distance rule, is an emergency, such as relieving a burn or wound, in which case the light may be a shorter distance, about 18 inches, for a more laser effect.

Most schedules contain a short series of colors. For instance, here's one that I personally use. Arthritis, which is Green, Magenta, then Blue. Notice the *function* of the colors are Green (stimulating muscle and tissue), Magenta (stimulating blood circulation), and the Blue (removing inflammation). It is important that they are used in the sequence given because they act like gears, shifting the gears of healing. Within the color spectrum, there are stimulating, relaxing, and neutral or balancing colors.

Allow about 20 minutes for each color, but even five minutes is beneficial. I often use them while at my desk, and once I used them in the hospital to speed my recovery. Since this process works gradually, several sessions may be required. It's not necessary to remove any clothing during a *tonation*, or to be in a dark room. It can be done any time of the day or night, but it's recommended to avoid stimulating colors before you sleep.

Color light therapy should be one of our first lines of defense, and can assist other modalities. It has prolonged effects, and can be used for extreme conditions and emotional and mental health. It greatly accelerates detoxification, making it ideal for obesity and breaking substance abuse.

Currently, in the U. S., color light therapy is approved for veterinarian use, and is increasingly popular for pets. Bear in mind that pets and children are more sensitive so the light and shorter sessions are recommended.

In this age of increasing diseases, remember that light therapy can penetrate beyond the effects of some other therapies, and can significantly increase healing.

I will share my first-hand color light experiences, one which was actually healing *in my hand.* I had a severe cut on my thumb, and several months later, I could still feel nerve pain traveling through my hand. Physical therapy helped some, but I still had daily pain. I began bathing my hand in turquoise light (a combination of relaxing blue and balancing green) for 20 minutes. During the first session, I felt a light electrical sensation, like the electric stem machine produces in the deep tissue. Then, during the next session, I felt a light throbbing, as when blood is circulating. On the third day, the pain greatly diminished, after almost a whole year! At this moment, I received my personal reward for months of research, and soon, my son did too. He had a fall that skinned a large patch on his arm with protruding blood tissue. As I ran to the store for more first aid supplies, I put the turquoise light on his arm, and by the time I returned in thirty minutes, he said, "Mom, it worked! My arm doesn't hurt anymore!" Case closed!

Another testimony was with diverticulosis. I had been hospitalized. Then I began the light schedule for diverticulosis (green, lemon, yellow and indigo), and within two hours, I began to feel relief. I continued this schedule at home, and within four days, my stools finally returned completely normal (after two months).

Learning and properly applying the science of color medicine has a rainbow of possibilities. It is so simple that anyone can learn and apply this with almost miraculous results. Shouldn't this one also be a part of every medical professional's repertoire, and in every home?

Eat the Rainbow

Now that we have seen the dazzling curative *healing* power of colors, let's look on the other side of the rainbow, at the health benefits of each color. As Ghadiali and others grasped the rainbows healing *rays*, so we can consume the rainbow's healthy *arrays, to* color your plate in a way that makes you thrive.

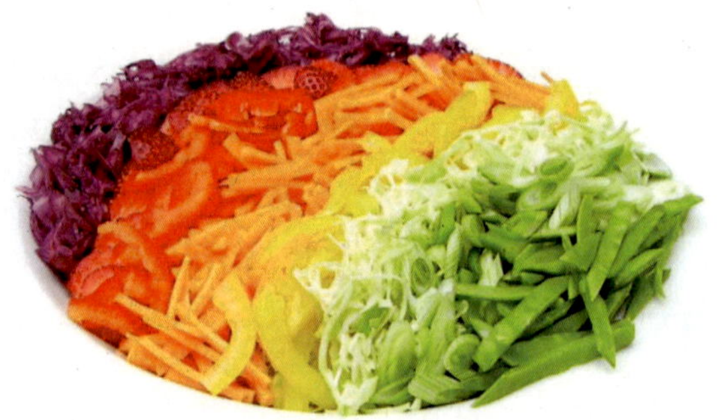

Color coded benefits of Fruits and Vegetables

Vegetables and fruits in a variety of colors provide the best all-around health benefits. Each color has unique essential qualities in nutrient rich whole foods.

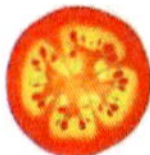

Reds (the color of the heart and blood) Helps keep your heart strong, reduces the risk of cancer, and lowers blood pressure.

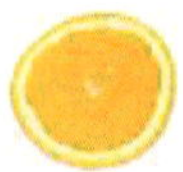

Orange / Yellow (the base color of skin) Improves skin quality and promotes collagen formation, healthy joints, and eyes.

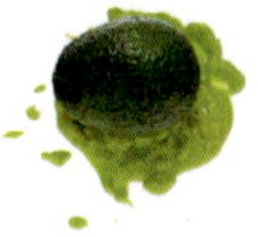

Green vegetables and fruit (the color of spring regeneration) Mineral rich support of bones, teeth, retinal health and digestion; boosts immunity; and creates mental energy and creativity.

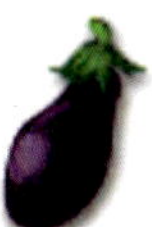

Blue and purple fruits and vegetables protects and supports mental and retinal health, reduces inflammation, boosts immune system, supports digestion, improves mineral absorption, and lowers inflammation.

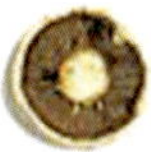

White fruits and vegetables reduces the risk of colon and hormone-related cancers, and balances hormone levels.

Green	White	Red	Yellow/Orange	Blue/Purple
Asparagus	Bananas	Beets	Apricots	Black currants
Avocados	Brown pears	Cherries	Butternut squash	Black salsify
Broccoli	Cauliflower	Cranberries	Cantaloupe	Blackberries
Celery	Dates	Guava	Carrots	Blueberries
Cabbage	Garlic	Papaya	Golden kiwifruit	Dried plums
Cucumbers	Ginger	Pink grapefruit	Lemon	Eggplant
Endive	Jerusalem artickoke	Pomegranates	Mangoes	Elderberries
Green apples	Mushrooms	Radicchio	Nectarines	Grapes
Green beans	Onions	Radishes	Oranges	Plums
Green grapes	Parsnips	Raspberries	Papayas	Pomegranates
Green onion	Potatoes	Red apples	Peaches	Prunes
Green pears	Shallots	Red chili peppers	Pineapples	Purple Belgian endive
Honeydew	Turnips	Red grapes	Pumpkin	Purple Potatoes
Kiwifruit	White Corn	Red onions	Sweet corn	Purple asparagus
Leafy greens	White nectarines	Red pears	Sweet potatoes	Purple cabbage
Leeks	White peaches	Red peppers	Tangerines	Purple carrots
Lettuce		Red potatoes	Yellow apples	Purple figs
Limes		Rhubarb	Yellow pears	Purple grapes
Okra		Strawberries	Yellow peppers	Purple peppers
Spinach		Tomatoes	Yellow potatoes	Raisins
Peas		Watermelon	Yellow squash	
Zucchini			Yellow tomatoes	

Soul Reflection of the Rainbow

Color is an amazingly powerful element in God's creation. It can effectively improve our physical environment, enhance our mental projection, provide deeper meaning in meditation, and add new dimensions to prayer. We can formulate powerful imagery that builds faith, just as God showed Abraham images in the sky above and in the sand at his feet. Below are the soul meanings of the rainbow colors, which can portray picturesque prayer and positive images.

RED is the stimulating and intense color of love, passion, and individuality. It is the color of the fire in our aspirations, sexuality, and the energy to express our unique qualities. As the color of the root chakra, it is our soul generator. When red is mixed with white (the color of purity), it becomes pink, the gentle, tender power of love. Usage: Add a little red in your environment or visualize in prayer someone surrounded by red roses for those needing inspiration for their aspirations; and picture pink roses around the rigid *ice queen* in your life and see what happens!

ORANGE is the stimulating (though less intensive) color of joy, creativity, and sociability. It is the playful color of a child; it encourages creativity and joyful play in adults as well as social engagement. Since orange is the color for the digestive chakra, there is a natural link: eating should be joyful and social. Usage: Decorate in orange to bring these qualities into your home, office, or facility. (I intuitively chose orange for my office walls before I knew the meaning of orange.) Pray for someone needing these attributes surrounded by orange blooms of spring iris.

YELLOW is the brightest color, like the sun, and is associated with intellectual brightness and cheerfulness. In the intellectual process, however, there is a natural tendency for personal distance to allow for objectivity, innovation, originality, and change - follow yellow. Yellow is fresh air, spring flowers, and cleansing. As the color of the solar-plexus chakra, it is the communicator between intuition and thoughts. Yellow reflects the analytical mind, and deep yellow (gold) reflects wisdom. Usage: Accessorize with yellow stimulus in schools, daycares, offices, or set bright sunflowers around someone needing these qualities.

GREEN is the center color of the rainbow and is our color for grounding, centering, and springtime renewal. Green is neutral, neither stimulating nor relaxing, creating balance in the body and mind, and therefore mirrors health and healing. The strong cleansing effect of green strengthens and stabilizes the nervous system and the entire body. When the heart chakra is balanced (green), one's whole life can flourish. Usage: Imagine how our creator placed us in the midst of a garden filled with greenery! What an amazing color to allow us to flourish! Perhaps that's where we need to spend more time,to be balanced, find our well-being, and get rejuvenated. What a great place to visualize someone you're praying for, in a lush green garden, surrounded by the preferred color of flowers.

BLUE skies are the earth's natural dome of light. It is the color of relaxation and growth. Plants flourish under blue lights, as do human cells. Is it any wonder why all of life was placed under this blue dome? Blue relaxes our heart and helps us breathe deeper, thereby receiving quality oxygen. (Blue is also associated with oxygen.) Blue reduces stress and anxiety, providing a feeling of heavenly peace. Usage: Blue is the color for the third-eye-chakra, or the forehead, which is where we usually feel stress and headache. Lots of blue in our lives can be ours just by basking outside on a blue skies day. And that's a great meditation.

TURQUOISE combines green and blue, becoming regenerating and relaxing. Turquoise is cooling and refreshing, and is therefore a primary anti-inflammatory color, which also has an emotional quality, supporting both our bodily and emotional healing. It powerfully relaxes irritated nerves. It removes the sting of even the worst burns in a short time. Usage: As the throat chakra, turquoise is the color for the thymus gland supporting the immune system. Our immunity is optimized when inflammation is removed. Turquoise Hydrangea - what a lovely flower to plant in your refreshing prayer garden!

VIOLET blends red and blue, which relates to activity and relaxation. It expresses respect and dignity towards oneself, others, and spiritual connection, reflecting a deep knowledge and understanding of harmony in relationships. It elevates us to our higher dreams, missions, and callings. Usage: Violet is the color for the crown chakra, the top of our head. It crowns us with value and honor and has a high vibration to propel into our spiritual destination. What a royal color to wrap around someone in your prayers.

Spiritual Reflection of the Rainbow Light

The Lord has provided colors to rejuvenate, soothe, and balance our body and soul. He has also arched a rainbow of colorful nutrition in our food that we may live our *full* life, *fully* alive.

As we have seen, the *rainbow* is so much more than the Lord's covenant to never again flood the earth. It is also His blessing *to flood* the earth with restorative, peaceful, balancing, and rejuvenating colors for complete healing and health. It is His mighty bow of mercy, expressing The Lord's intense compassion with a penetrating arrow of light.

He calls us "children of light." As color emanates from natural light, so we become the colors of the spiritual light. We bear His same essence, reflected in many hues. We are each a unique expression of the Lord in full living color: soothing, calming, inspiring, reviving, strengthening, regenerating, stabilizing, creating, and re-creating. We are vibrant, as our light glows in true full colors! May we shine our light boldly, like Dr. Dinshah and Dr. Kate, leaving a colorful legacy and finishing the race strong! The first chapter of *In the Light* portrays the heroic story of Dr. Dinshah as an outstanding warrior of the Lord who continually battled the forces of darkness with light and love. He continued his ministry of compassion and wisdom with perseverance and ingenuity, building a solid foundation of healing for present and future generations, in spite of continual unbearable persecution. He truly was the unstoppable light that is still prevailing against darkness and disease today!

Health Coach Recommendations

1. Eat an array of colors of whole foods daily, since each has different nutritional contributions.
2. Eat plenty of the color you need, such as reds for heart or blood issues.
3. Create a supportive living environment with colors that enhance in areas where you work, play, or sleep, such as orange to inspire creativity, yellow for intellectual stimulation, or blue for soothing.
4. Notice what colors you are drawn to and what it reveals about you.
5. Use colors in mental imagery to change your mood, meditate, or pray. Green is the color of balance, which can help put us back in balance.
6. Consider learning and using color therapy for your own healing and others. Kits and classes can be ordered from www.coloredlighttherapy.com. Or you can build your own as per instructions by the Dinshah Health Society in *Let there be Light*.

Recommended Readings

Let There Be Light by Darius Dinshah
Color Medicine by Charles Klotsche
Change Your Life With The Secret Power of Color
by Martin Kutternick and Colin G. Smith

May the rainbow color our lives, inspire creativity, heal our ailments, maintain balance, and fully express our passion, character, and values. Surely it delights our Heavenly Father when we cherish this beautiful gift for our enjoyment and health, just as when our children enjoy the gifts we give. How much more, our Heavenly Father?

We now conclude Part 1 with caring for the vital part of being, our etheric (auric) body, our energy and soul life (not to be confused with the imperishable spirit of man).

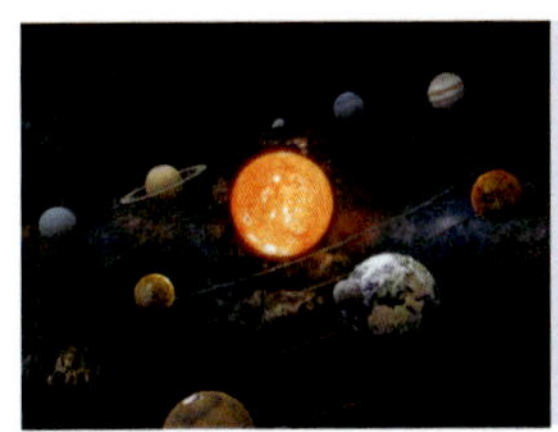

Chapter 4

The Healing Power of Sound

"And God said..." (Genesis 1:3).

At the sound of God's voice, our Creator's power was released and the universe came into existence. Science has revealed that we can hear the resulting echoes of the amazing birth of creation called *Cosmic Background Radiation*, first discovered in 1965 by Nobel Prize winning scientist, George Smoot, who said, "[It] is like seeing the face of God." (See: http://www.physics.org/featuredetail.asp?id=45)

Envision the Lord's voice resounding in vibratory motion through all of creation. As His vibrational healing power surges through us when we attune our energy system to proper *light waves*, so there is also restorative wholeness when we align with nature's *sound waves.* Like musical instruments, we are somewhat dysfunctional when *out of tune*, but become healthier and harmonized when aligned with our natural design. We, too, can be *finely tuned* for our best emotional and physical wellbeing.

"Every cell in our body is a sound resonator. Every cell lives in a dynamic rhythmic pattern. Each organ has its own cycle and its own pulse. Each and every system has a cycle, rhythm, pattern, and pulse that exist in resonant harmony and sympathy to the cycles of the earth and the heavens. These body systems respond to sound vibration, as do our spiritual, mental, and emotional states of consciousness." (Donna Carey, Lac)

Everything in the Universe is vibrating; from planets and stars to the smallest particles, including the human body, all are creating sound wave patterns. We are in constant vibration and every organ and tissue in our bodies has its own specific rate of vibration, as does each chakra and layer of our electromagnetic field or *aura*. Sound therapy is based on the principle of one vibrating object causing another to vibrate in harmony with it by matching its rate of vibration. This is how the powerful voice of an opera singer can break glass with the sheer power of vocal chords (and strong lungs), or how the low vibrations of a passing truck may rattle your trinkets.

Since every part of the body and its associated magnetic field is vibrating, then each part of the body, whether an organ or chakra, must have its optimum healthy frequency. Thus, illness may result when some part of us is not vibrating harmoniously as we were designed. The afflicted parts can be supported by directing the correct sound frequency that promotes the optimum, healthy vibration. Sound therapy essentially re-tunes the body-mind, allowing the body to restore itself. It nurtures the nervous system, calms emotions, reduces pain, alleviates stress, and improves focus and general wellbeing. How is this achieved?

Harmonious Vibrations can be used to create mental and bodily wellness by simply listening to specific frequencies of sound. Notice that the same polar opposites of light correspond with sound, varying from stimulating, balancing, to relaxing colors; so sound projects certain frequencies influencing all areas of our health, including mental and emotional states as seen in the range of sound waves below:

gamma	inspiration	higher learning	focus
beta	alertness	concentration	cognition
alpha	relaxation	visualization	creativity
theta	meditation	intuition	memory
delta	healing	sleep	detached awareness

The *Gamma* brain wave phase occurs in accelerated intellectual or athletic peaks, while *Beta* reflects our normal cognitive state of alertness. *Alpha* brings calm relaxation, cultivating creativity and visualization, and releasing stress for the ideal condition before engaging in life's challenges. *Theta*, the semi-conscious state prior to deep sleep, is the first level of healing that recharges the immune system. Finally, *Delta* is the state of deep sleep that includes the regeneration of cellular level healing.

The various sound vibrations are similar to light *gears*, in that they help us transcend from the beta level to specific levels of healing, creativity and awareness. Within a short time, the body absorbs and matches the proper frequency, resulting in desired results such as accelerated recovery, enhanced growth hormone levels, and sound sleep.

Healing with sound waves or vibrations is a natural healing modality that has been used successfully since ancient medicine. Brass healing bowls, gongs, and bells created harmonious healing energy to bringing back natural healthy balance in all bodily systems. Musical instruments create vibrations that help bring the heart and mind back into balance.

We may not always be aware of how music and sounds impacts our feelings, but they are significantly influencing our health whether we realize it or not. According to the National Institutes of Health (NIH), studies show that certain music can reduce pain, blood pressure, anxiety, and ease depression (NIH, 2010). Sound Healing is an established health profession, using a variety of sounds, gongs, bowls, music, etc. It can be used alone or combined with other therapies like massage, acupuncture, and light therapy!

Consider how most children are quite responsive to sound and music and are naturally creative. Certified Cross-Cultural Music Healing Practitioner, Loretta Brown, tells of her fascination with sound which began when she was three years old. "I discovered I could imitate the sound of thunder on the low notes of the piano and the rain on the high notes. The sound was already speaking to me, and for years I searched for a way to utilize sound and music in healing."

Benefits of Sound Healing:

- Reduces stress and anxiety
- Improves concentration
- Enhances creativity
- Improves vision in all spheres
- Balances brain hemisphere
- Stabilizes hormonal balance
- Relieves sinus congestion and headaches
- Increases energy
- Cleanses and balances Chakras and the aura
- Stimulates intuition

In a 2009 article published by The National Center for Biotechnology Information (NCBI), Dr. Assad Meymandi writes: "Since ancient times, music has been recognized for its therapeutic value. Greek physicians used flutes, lyres, and zithers to heal their patients. *They used vibration to aid in digestion, treat mental disturbance, and induce sleep.* Aristotle (373–323 BCE), in his famous book *De Anima*, wrote that flute music could arouse strong emotions and purify the soul. Ancient Egyptians describe musical incantations for healing the sick."

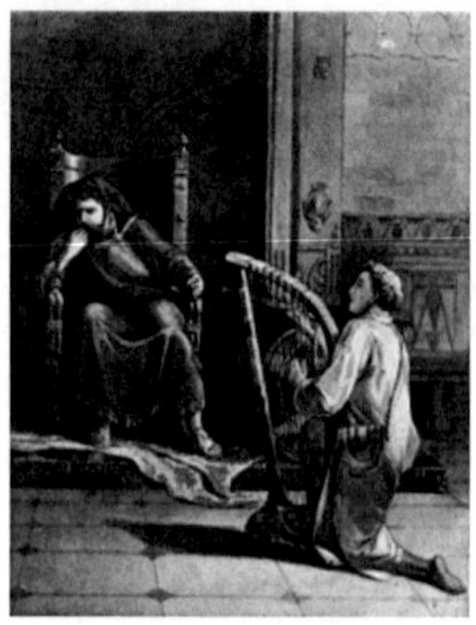

King David soothed King Saul with the healing sounds of his lyre.

Modern Uses of Sound Therapy

The concert of the universe is merged into health care through the use of precision-calibrated planetary *tuning forks* and symphonic *planetary gongs*. Acupressure points and chakras provide non-invasive access into our core bodily energy systems. This natural healing art is called *Acutonics,* a non-invasive practice that integrates well into clinical practices such as physicians, nurses, acupuncturists, massage, chiropractors, psychologists, physical therapists, energy medicine practitioners, and many other health care providers. *Medicinal music* is used in hospitals to soothe postoperative pain, lower blood pressure, and boost immunity. Like light therapy, there are many methods of reaping the benefits of sound.

Musical CDs, set to specific healing and inspirational tones, are simple, convenient ways that can be used anywhere, any time. A most profound product is called "Wholetones" by renowned musician, author and speaker, Michael Tyrrell. He first explains frequencies by giving the example that a *frequency* is created when you speak. Your voice box vibrates, and when you form words your tongue vibrate-like the ones your voice box and tongue make every day. *These frequencies,* he explains, *have the divine power to heal you.* He presents his music therapy through a series of CDs (or downloads) which can be ordered at wholetones.com (at a very reasonable cost).

Below, he shares his amazing insights and story, revealing his stunning discovery of 7 musical tones that relieve stress, promote healing, break negative cycles, and restore sound sleep:

- We identify frequencies using a unit of measurement called *Hertz*. Hertz measures sound as 1 vibrational cycle per second.
- In ancient times, at least 7 of these frequencies were used to heal and protect…recorded in 7 songs…I call it *Wholetones: The Healing Frequency Music Project…*

- I was given a very special gift that I'm going to share with you (regarding)…ancient frequencies that I believe were played by King David himself – to heal and soothe King Saul in his time of depression. These ancient healing frequencies are so powerful, the Lord told me to create a product...so He could give these frequencies back to us – and everyone could experience their amazing power, recorded in 7 songs...I call… *Wholetones: The Healing Frequency Music Project…*(the) '7 Secret Frequencies Uncovered in the Music of King David'.

Here's (the) synopsis of (this) powerful, creative modality of health…simply by listening daily to this music:

1. Wipe out … unhealthy fears … guilt and shame, and help(s) restore…liver, brain, and kidney functions...(SONG 1, 396Hz)
2. Remove the recurring negative cycles … procrastination, addiction, and junk food...as sluggishness and lethargy disappear and productivity and creativity increase...enhance digestion, ease stomach issues, balance metabolism, erase headaches and … back pain...(SONG 2 417Hz)
3. Discover the Master Key that precipitates all other frequencies. You'll feel soothed by its multiple health benefits as you're tenderly enveloped in peace. This is the very same frequency David used to soothe King Saul's depression... (SONG 3, 444Hz)
4. Hear the most curious frequency of all...it has the power to relax you...transform your stress into peaceful bliss. Creating the ideal environment for your body to repair hormonal imbalances, ease muscle tension, and release troubles of circulation...(SONG 4, 528Hz)
5. Enjoy the fostering of peace and forgiveness in all your relationships. Also known to positively affect the endocrine system – particularly gall bladder and adrenal issues... (SONG 5, 639Hz)
6. Gain a keen awareness of your very own spirit in this powerful yet delicately performed miracle of healing. Experience deep spiritual and emotional healing, while

cleansing your immune system of common infections. Super-charge your circulatory system to support your healthy heart and blood flow...(SONG 6, 741Hz)

7. 7. Revel in the frequency that celebrates the King of Kings. Purely spiritual – connect in the worship of God, His love for humankind, and His return to those who await Him... (SONG 7, 852Hz)

I have *a rather unusual story* to quickly share, so you understand the power of this project and how it came to life.

This divine gift I'm sharing with you today was given to me while I was in Jerusalem...I met a piano player…in Jerusalem who changed my life...a mysterious but wonderful Christian piano player named David (of course!) who was performing Christian songs of worship – in a Jewish Orthodox coffee house!

He noticed that I was aware of what he was doing...and smiled at me – he knew I was a believer. On a break, he ran to his car, came back, and sat down next to me. *What happened next changed my life forever ...*

David's life's work was studying the ancient psalms of King David – in ancient Hebraic forms of music...and he handed me manuscript copies of many of these psalms. He then said – 'These are for you…Yeshua said you would know what to do with them.'

Well, let me tell you – both of us wept!

Sometime later, I looked at one of the manuscripts and noticed something mysterious...David had adapted them to a modern key. Sonically – this simply didn't work. So I reflected on our conversation that night in Jerusalem... 'Yeshua said you would know what to do with them.'

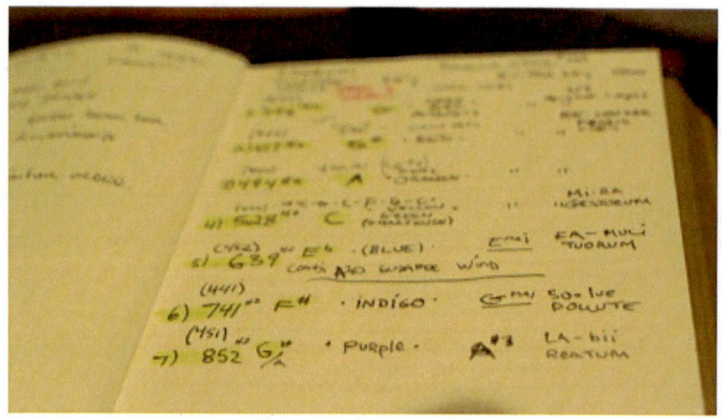

The manuscript of healing

Suddenly...the light came on...I DID know what to do!

I noticed *the original manuscript was in a different key...* supposedly, *King* David tuned his instruments higher than what we know as the *modern musical tuning system.* I decided to experiment. I found reference to King David in my Bible on page *222.*

Now I don't know if this was divine intervention or not, but something told me to double that page number and re-tune my guitar..."That's when I realized...*I think I just discovered the key of David.* So I quickly grabbed my guitar and tuned it up to 444 hertz. Remember: Hertz measures sound as 1 vibrational cycle per second – these are frequencies...that each sound vibrates 444 times per second.

Once I re-tuned, I discovered that most of these ancient healing frequencies were now right under my fingers. And I'm convinced that God had given these frequencies to King David, and I know for a fact that my piano playing friend David gave them to me.

Some listeners have reported almost automatic healing...one in as little as 22 minutes!

...My mom was diagnosed with pancreatic cancer in 2005. And they said she'd need a 4-hour surgery to remove the tumor. Of course my wife and I made a mad-dash to be there with her. ...*I brought my guitar along with our bags.* The night before she was to go to the operating room, I asked my mom if she would like me to play for her. She readily agreed.

I tuned my guitar and began playing in the 741Hz frequency...I gently placed the headstock of the instrument on her side...approximating the location of her pancreas.

As my mom recalls,

Michael felt like the Lord would have him play his guitar over me and I was more than willing.

He said for me just to close my eyes – and I did – As I did that, I don't remember...I asked him how long afterwards... did he play and he said approximately 20 minutes. I don't remember that at all-all I remember is when I closed my eyes, probably 2 or 3 minutes after my eyes were closed I could see this...this thing... this black, round looking thing with tentacles and I just kept my eyes closed and as he played and played that mass that I assumed was what they'd seen on their diagnostic test in me, is what I was seeing in my mind's eye. It began to fade.

And it got less and less dark... and all of the sudden – everything went green. And it was the brightest green I ever saw in my life. And I said I'm healed ...

When it was time for her to have her operation, we were told they'd be in for about 4 hours, but mom and I both knew that she was already healed. Still, they took her in, but then something wonderful happened ...

After 45 minutes the surgeon came in beaming – 'No cancer! no cancer!...everything is clear!'

In fact, just before the surgeon came busting in with the good news...right after the nurse told us he'd be in to speak with us, I said, "She's healed. The cancer is gone." And I was right. My mother is still tumor-free...9 years later!

I believe these frequencies were passed down to King David by God Himself. His original manuscripts were transcribed by my dear friend – an amazing piano player and believer – David from Jerusalem. He gave me these manuscripts and when I took a closer look, I understood they were transcribed to A=440 Hz which was inconsistent with what I knew of King David's tuning. I sought to "right the wrong" and re-tuned my guitar to match King David's original frequency. By divine intervention all this led to the creation of... *The Wholetones Healing Frequency Music Project.*

Truthfully we had no idea what we were going to play when we went into the studio...This further affirms to us that God was conducting this project from its humble start to the glorious finish. We used the best gear we could find. We recorded the music with analog technology where possible with minimal digital sampling. We used the finest instruments...crafted from the finest materials. When we started playing, we all simultaneously felt the hand of God guide us through each song...in the end, it's the healing frequencies that matter – the music is merely the vehicle."

Indeed, the voice of God ripples with healing waves throughout His creation. "*...the mountains and hills will burst into song before you, and all the trees of the field will clap their hands*" (Isaiah 55:12). We too can be finely tuned by this glorious Genesis gem!

Recommended Reading:

Wholetones by Michael Tyrrell
Tuning the Human Biofield: Healing with Vibrational Sound Therapy by Eileen Day McKusick

Health Coach Recommendations:

- Play healing tones wherever possible: home, office, travel, and outdoors
- Consider *Acutonics* as a natural healing remedy.
- Combine Sound Therapy with other modalities such as Light Therapy or massage.

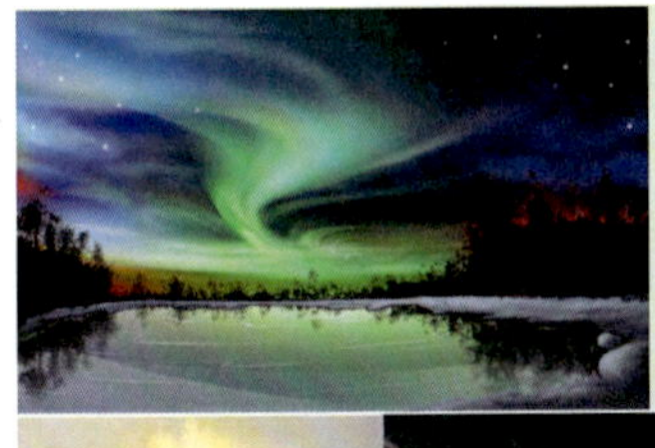

Chapter 5

Nourishing the Etheric body

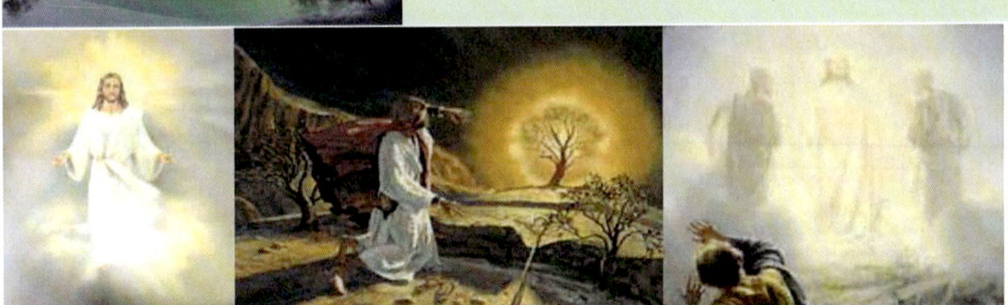

We have seen how light, color, and sleep attunes our etheric energy system to receive wholeness and healing. Now, let's take a step back, and clearly define the etheric (auric) body. What makes it thrive; and what makes it dive, so to speak?

We must first explore the Genesis foundational gift of light, before discussing terms such as chakra, etheric energy, and auric views, which may be questionable in mainstream Christianity. Yet, consider these biblical and scientific views that will help us clearly see the light.

Auric light (or auric darkness) is simply the manifestation of the light or darkness emanating from a being or object. This is why when God or Jesus was manifest in various forms, such as the burning bush, on Mt. Sinai, in the transfiguration, at Jesus' resurrection, and in Paul's blinding confrontation and the many angelic appearances, there appears intense, often blinding light. Indeed, the light of the Lord is too overwhelming for the human eye and mind.

Yet, since we are created in His image, we too are surrounded by this same quality of light. Thus, we are called the children of light, and a light for others. God's word is called the light; and we manifest the light to the extent that His word abides in us. The auric quality of light surrounding us is manifest by our purity, as expressed in this excerpt from summitlighthouse.org

"The Aura of a Saint". (Remember that in the scriptures we too are called saints.)

"…Blessed are the pure in heart, for they shall see God." Not only shall they see God but they shall be (reflect) God. For the pure in heart—by purity of desire, motive, speech, conduct and works—continually qualify with light the stream of energy that flows through the heart. And that pure light fills the aura.

So, seeing God is possible because there is something within us that we can equate with God and thereby we can identify (with) God. That "something" is his light. God's light is his greatest gift to us. It is like water: it will take on the color, the vibration, the density that we put upon it. We can change water from a liquid to ice or vapor.

God's light is our immediate resource, and it is continually flowing like liquid, like moving fire…"

Think of etheric energy like electricity; and electricity can be used for good or evil. It can provide energy to preserve us, or it can destroy life. While this gift might be used for evil, we can glorify God by using it for His healing power, as set forth in these chapters on light and color light. Wouldn't it make sense that the "father of lies" would steer us away from using this marvelous gift of light by drawing our attention to how it is used for ungodly purposes? Therefore, let your conclusion be filtered through the light of God's word."

So don't be misled, my dear brothers and sisters. Whatever is good and perfect comes down to us from God our Father, who created all the lights in the heavens. He never changes or casts a shifting shadow. (James 1:16, 17 NLT)

Since light, and color light energy heals us perfectly and precisely through our etheric being, shouldn't we embrace this enlightening gift of creation?

Our Etheric body is like our human electrical system with numerous energy networks called nadis or meridians. Where streams of energy meet and cross, from the base of the spine to the crown of the head, they create major energy channels called Chakras. Chakras are aligned with the endocrine glands (glands producing hormones that regulate metabolism, growth and development, tissue function, sexual function, etc.). This field of energy then radiates outward from the gateway center. There are also 21 minor energy centers throughout the body, with powerful energy points located in the arms and hands.

One day, I asked The Lord to show me my own auric shell. Later that day, I had a thought to stare at my arm (against the background wall), continuously with a peripheral vision, and move it very slowly. Within a few minutes, I could clearly see a blue border, about one inch surrounding my arm.

The *quality* of our physical body and soul is reflected in our etheric body. The etheric state can even be detected in subliminal odors. A spiritually whole person disperses a pleasant odor, such as the scriptures refer to "the sweet smell of Christ." In contrast, one who is consumed by evil protrudes a subtle scent of decay, as Christ called, *a foul spirit.* (Of course, this refers to one's spiritual, not physical, body odor.)

A healthy body and soul projects rays that are clear and rigid, whereas the lines are droopy and lifeless in bodies affected by disease. *Disease and illness often begin by the degeneration of the etheric body and later manifests in the physical.* For instance, chronic stress is even recognized in the Western world to be the primary *cause* of most diseases. The great news is that you can master your soul life *with a double* benefit of increasing the body's ability to heal and slow the aging process.

The primary way we nurture our etheric body is with positive light, both natural sunlight and positive emotions. Positive thoughts and feelings uphold and strengthen this vital part of us, while the negative weakens it. These two polar energies, the positive or negative, each have magnetic forces which draw in more of the same, as we'll see how to harness this energy in the Law of Attraction.

For instance, positive meditation such as prayer, combined with the full spectrum of light (natural sunlight) generates healing in all chakras. This elevates self-healing abilities and the positive vibrational energy that protect us from the negative. On the other side, anxiety, worry, and fear cause congestion at the etheric level. Here is where we must seriously consider blocking internal and external dark influences, because they deplete *irreplaceable* etheric energy. Guard your heart with a protective wall against negativity.

There are also other factors that fortify etheric energy such as the quality of food (eat organic when possible), water, and air. Foods high in etheric energy are meats (from naturally grazed animals) and (moderately) cooked vegetables. While cooking destroys some nutrients, it raises the etheric energy. Fresh foods grown in nutrient rich soil are best, since food loses this energy after a while.

Additionally, drinking pure spring water, breathing oxygen-rich air, getting adequate sleep and rest, and keeping your physical body warm, all help conserve this energy.

An array of natural healing arts can relieve energy blocks and rejuvenate the flow, such as chiropractic care, acupuncture, and massage. Various stretching practices such as Yoga and Tai Chi balance and energize the etheric body. Detoxifying and toning the liver and other organs increases their ability to absorb more etheric energy.

Finally, modern technology has filled our atmosphere with electromagnetic pollution for communication networks and electronic appliances, causing *electromagnetic stress*, resulting in headaches, fatigue, bad moods, and potentially, disease. While there's not much we can do about the world we live in, we can do our best to minimize and distance ourselves from this interference. Mobile phones, for example, have high levels of interference that strain the body.

Over time, this strain can greatly impact our bodies. For

instance, a study of men who continuously wear their phones on one side showed a significant *softness in bone density on the side that they carry their phone*. While we can't toss away our phones, we can at least try to keep them at a distance when possible.

Dr. Lawrence Wilson advises that we were born with a certain amount of etheric energy, and that by preserving it, we maintain the quality and quantity of our life. One of the keys to longevity is conserving it with these recommendations.

Health Coach Recommendations

- Press the delete button on negativity, and capture positive light (thoughts).
- Meditation and prayer help us to be more optimistic and ease stress.
- Eat quality food, and drink pure spring water
- Deeply breathe oxygen-rich air when possible
- Get adequate sleep and rest, and keep your physical body comfortably warm
- Rejuvenate the energy flow by healing arts and energizing exercise
- Distance yourself from electronics when possible. Place your mobile phone as far from your body as is reasonable. Keep distance from microwaves, too.

Spiritual Reflection of Etheric Body

Since the etheric body exists in the less tangible sphere, much like electricity, we tend to be unconscious of it until there's interference. Once we lose the power in our home, however, we suddenly realize how many things run on electricity. Suddenly, almost everything becomes non-functional!

So it is with this less visible, but dominant part of our being (like our spirit). When we nourish our spirit, we quicken our mortal bodies. When we nourish our etheric bodies, we enrich our physical body and spiritual being. The same self-care that is good for the physical body is also good for the etheric, as we have been created as a harmonious masterpiece!

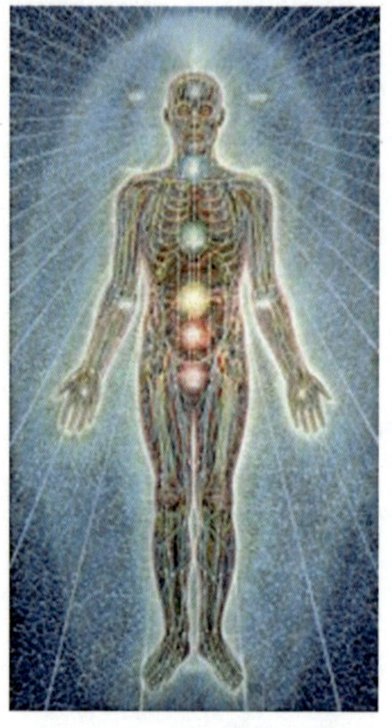
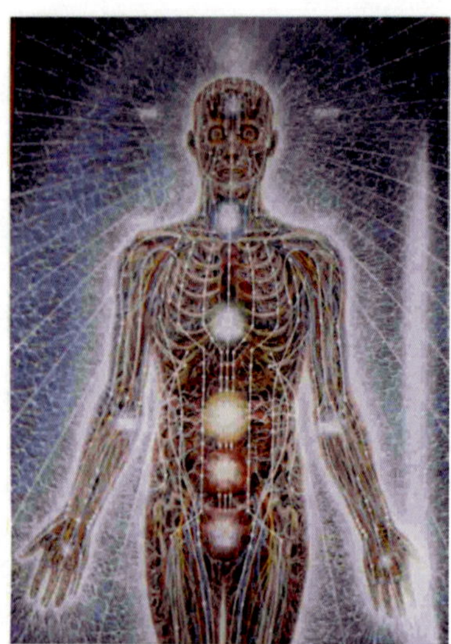

Notice the fine webbing of the etheric body crossing in the center, creating major energy hubs, much like major airport networks.

See the minor energy centers located in the arm and hands? When we stretch forth our hands to heal, embrace someone, massage, or simply touch, we are releasing etheric energy that reaches beyond the skin, into the soul. Through our elaborate channels, natural energy flows in *laying on of hands* and touching others.

What an amazing *Designer* who created us with a self-re-charging battery source that regulates and re-boots its *double.* Every energy point is intricately and perfectly placed within the human body to harness balance, that it can continually restore and heal itself.

Caring for the etheric body enhances self-care for the physical body, where we'll now see how your genetic makeup determines the best foods, exercise, and self-care for YOU.

Part 2

Physical Nutrition

(genetic design)

"One man's food is another man's poison."

You could view a hundred healthy lifestyle websites and see a hundred different opinions defining healthy foods, exercise, and self-care. Some authorities advise vegetarian, while others meat; some say milk, and others - no dairy. Some recommend wheat, or not. Amidst all the confusion, you say, "I'll just eat what I *feel* like eating."

Now you begin to arrive at the moment of truth - because what your mammal instinct intuitively *tells you* to eat is the ultimate authority on health and nutrition. It is not what our minds tell us to eat, but rather, what our body truly directs. Unfortunately, over time, we may have been so confused by dietary theories and advertisement of unhealthy food that we've lost touch with our inner captain. You may find your *best genetic foods* right in your freezer that you chose *intuitively*, as I did, before I learned about eating and exercising in harmony with my own genetics, such as my blood and body types.

For each blood type, some foods are compatible while others are incompatible; even some *healthy* foods are not well-suited for your type and should be *avoided*. Dr. James D'Adamo, author of *Eat Right For(4) Your Type* speaks of the individuality of blood types.

"I believed that no two people on the face of the earth were alike; no two people have the same fingerprints, lip prints, or voiceprints. No two blades of grass or snowflakes are alike. Because I felt that all people were different from one another, I did not think it was logical that they should eat the same foods.

It became clear to me that since each person was housed in a special body with different strengths, weaknesses, and nutritional requirements, the only way to maintain health or cure illness was to accommodate to the particular patient's specific needs."

Dr. Joseph Christiano, author of *Blood types Body types and You*, shares his perspective, that we are each "custom built", according to our genetic foundation.

"You are what you eat, but it is also vitally important for you to eat what you are! Your body type – or body genetics – is the foundation of the 'house' that is you, but custom building requires that you understand what strategies or building plans will work the best."

Let us now crack the code of your blood and body types as we wade through the science of anthropology and human genetics.

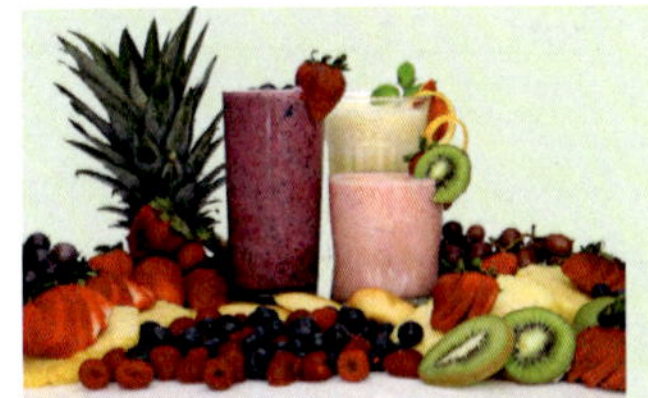

Chapter 6
Best Lifestyle for Your Blood Type

...for the life of the body is in its blood... (Lev. 17:11 NLT).

As food is assimilated, it transcends into the quality of our cells, blood, and even our thoughts! Therefore, consuming foods that are compatible with our blood type enhances the quality of our lives in every way.

Our genetic blueprint is engraved in our ancestral heritage. This is apparent when seeing our physical and emotional features mirrored in our children. Yet this branding penetrates far deeper than meets the eye. Our ancient ancestors leave a lasting impression, even in our blood.

By our genetic makeup, modern science can predict our vulnerabilities. A healthy lifestyle, in harmony with your blood type will help to protect you from your inherent weaknesses and strengthen your immunity and digestive ability. We will see this in great detail within each food category. Thus, there is no right or wrong diet, only the best choices according to your blood type.

Our body is guarded with *secret service agents* that create antibodies to foreign *antigens* (a chemical response) that tag it for destruction. This reaction is called *agglutination*, which literally glues them together, causing bacteria, virus, and parasites to stick and clump together for easy disposal – just like Spiderman does! Some blood types have more astringent secret service agents, and other types have more friendly security systems. (Agglutination can be seen on a short YouTube video: *Death by Sugar,* as processed sugar cause cells to clump together like caterpillars, slumping along.)

Beyond these obvious *bad guys,* like bacteria, are more subtle ones in foods called lectins (various proteins) that can have this agglutinating affect in our blood. Foods that are incompatible with your blood type also cause agglutination. We commonly call these allergies, sensitivities, or simply foods that *don't agree with us*. You may even recognize your blood type tendencies for certain disease or conditions.

This brief, simplified overview provides a visualization of what occurs within our delicate, intricate, internal *laboratory*. The full details are well explained in layman's terms in Dr. A'damo's, *Eat Right (4) Your Type*. Let's now see how and where each blood type evolved, and how we are enveloped in this unbroken *umbilical cord,* our blood type, which even reveals our personality traits.

Blood Type Development and Characteristics

Noah, a man of the soil, proceeded to plant a vineyard." (Genesis 9:20.) *He (Cush) was a mighty hunter before the Lord* (Genesis 10:8).

...the maritime peoples spread out into their territories, by their clans within their nations, each with its own language (Genesis 10:5).

According to Dr. A'damo, the human story of blood type evolution aligns with the biblical time frame. This development begins with the will to survive and, later, strategies to thrive – in search of food, cultivating food, or moving to find food (much like your hungry teenager). Here we begin the trail of survival.

After the flood, as we see in the scriptures above, Noah was "a man of the soil", and Cush was "a mighty hunter". Then there is migration "spreading out into their territories". When the hunters were exhausting their food source, they migrated from Africa to Europe and Asia, beginning a new food source - agriculture. Over time, as they traveled to cooler climates, they began to physically acclimatize with lighter skin, which provided more protection against frostbite and better metabolized vitamin D in lands with shorter days. Their hair also became straighter, a more adequate covering over their heads in frigid temperatures. Additionally, their eyes became lighter (such as blue and hazel), allowing greater night vision in climates with long nights, in contrast to darker skin and eyes which shield against the intense long sunlight hours.

Beyond these exterior genetic changes were also *internal* alterations as dietary changes impacted their digestibility and immunity, and even changing the *language* of their DNA, developing a new blood type. Like Star Wars shape-shifters, we became what we needed to be to survive. This is where blood type leaves its genetic fingerprint, with the qualities of ancestral type still running through our veins. *How genetically adaptable we have been created!*

Indeed, our blood retains a genetic memory engraved in a chain of generations. It has left a lasting impression on our ability to fend off infections and respond to stress. Blood type influences the immunity security in recognizing the good guys and killing off the bad guys. It has also left a footprint on the strength of the digestive process. This internal imprint is as viable as the external, such as eye and skin color.

Type "O" were skillful hunters, Cro-Magnons, appeared. These lean mean fighting machines could eat darned near everything – and probably did. Equipped with a high stomach acid, they probably crunched bones like potato chips. Their high protein diet kept these big boned beastly creatures ready for combat at any time.

Type "O" Profile

These traits still remain in those of us who share type "O," although you probably haven't wrestled for your game (unless you purchased your T-bone during a *bluelight special*). What remains, however, are these strong qualities:

- Meat eater with hardy digestion
- Overcharged immune system
- Stress response best with intense physical activity
- Thin blood prevents blood clotting and plaque artery build-up

These hardy blessings, however, also come with potential curses, although eating and exercising in harmony with your type can counteract these genetic tendencies. For instance, tendencies include ulcers due to strong stomach acid, arthritis due to overactive immune systems, and bleeding disorders due to thin blood. Additionally, Type "O"s tend to have unstable thyroids and a sluggish metabolism (a means of preservation during long periods with no catch). The Type "O" plan in the upcoming chapters will help you strategically overcome these pitfalls.

Blood type is also embedded in our personality traits. In fact, in some oriental cultures, blood type is a major component for career and mating compatibility. Type "O" is preferred for leadership or executive positions, while Type "A" makes a great social community coordinator. The same goes for what you're looking for in a spouse.

Ironically, the "O" blood type personality parallels the Myer-Briggs type "A." They are naturally the enduring, self-reliant, risk-taking, optimistic, healthy, focused, driven leadership kind. While these are inherent qualities, one's environment can, of course, alter the natural state. The upcoming lifestyle recommendations will help bring out your best, and most importantly, balance these polarities.

Type "A" Profile

"A" is Agrarian

Type "A" appeared in Asia or the Middle East when moving to a new environment with a new food supply – agriculture and animal domestication. They began to establish stable communities where they cultivated grains, other crops, and livestock. They traded in the spear for the spade. As they adapted to this new way of life, so did their biological responses. No longer needing a super digestion and immunity against wild predators, the strength of these processes decreased.

The greatest strength of type "A," however, is their adaptability to dietary and environmental changes. It is crucial that they use this to their advantage in combating the inherent weaknesses of sensitive digestion and vulnerable immunity. Type "A" has thicker blood, which has potential health risks. Type "A" also has a more delicate stress response which requires greater self-care. All of these factors combined have more genetic tendencies for serious disease. Self-care is of utmost importance for Type "A"; carefully considering everything from stress to diet and appropriate exercise. These precautions are presented in the next section. Contrary to Type "O," they thrive predominately on vegetarian protein with only certain small amounts of animal protein and gentle exercise.

The amazing character of Type A is reflected in an agriculture setting, and in a word: cooperative. Both farming and raising livestock requires flexibility, networking, and interactive skills for production. These traits still resonate in the type "A": teamwork, flexibility, orderly, respect for others, self-control, and cooperation. They flourish in community support and social activity.

Type "B" Profile

"B" is Balanced

Type "B" developed as tribes moved from eastern Africa to the Himalayan highlands (part of modern day Pakistan and India). There they became herdsman, dependent on domesticating animals, with a diet of cultured dairy and meat. As these nomads eventually moved toward Asia, some dispersed north and west, becoming hardy warriors and horsemen, and some settled in the south and east into an agrarian culture. This area, however, was not the ideal farmland, yet they created sophisticated irrigation and cultivation strategies that reflected their amazing creative intelligence.

The blood consistency of Type B is balanced between the thin ("O") and the thick ("A"), allowing more stability. They tolerate the greatest dietary variety, and are more durable in other ways, too. Type "B" shares many of the Type "O" *pros* and are more refined, therefore escaping some of the type "O" cons. You might think of "B" is for *blessed*, although this type has a few *odd* vulnerabilities too.

First, the strengths: overall balanced, strong immunity, tolerant digestive, with the most dietary variety, and a creative response to stress. Type "B"s are generally hardy and stable, but are more prone to less common conditions, such as multiple sclerosis, lupus, skin disorders, and chronic fatigue syndrome. Once again, abiding by their best blood type plan can help "B" be their *Best*.

Type "AB" Profile

"AB" is A Blend

The rare, Type "AB" emerged about a thousand years ago with a fusion of "A" and "B." Its genetic memory retains more of the hardy type "B" traits. It takes *good genes* from both *parents,* such as "A"s adaptability to environment and diet and "B"s enhanced immunity, inheriting the tolerance of both "A" and "B"; but it also includes the flaws of both, such as the Type "A" sensitive digestive tract. "AB" is a complex web of the strengths and weaknesses.

Type "AB" has tendencies for chemical imbalance disorders and hormonal imbalance. Women of this blood type have more potential for menstrual disorders. The general "AB" group is more predisposed to cancer, heart disease, anemia, and autoimmune disease. Nevertheless, this is where they can harness the optimistic values of their blend to support optimal health.

Summary of all Blood Types

As you see, each type is unique with its own blessings and curses. In the backdrop of this science is our core nature as mammals. In the animal kingdom, none is really superior, only different. Some thrive on intense physical activity, others, don't; some are carnivores, others not; and each innately cares for himself according to his design. As we learn to respond to our inner voice (beyond the social programming), we'll naturally position ourselves to better avoid disease, optimize energy, and acquire our ideal weight.

When we understand this aspect of our genetic design and of others it prepares us for a better quality of life, and greater longevity. It also helps us connect and build rapport with other blood type personalities as we truly understand *where they're coming from.* For instance, a Type "O" might appreciate the social skills or community contribution of a Type "A" and take care not to overwhelm their more delicate nervous system. A Type "A" might appreciate the leadership skills of a Type "O," and encourage their aspirations.

The following charts provide a brief summary of each type, including some dietary and supplement directives. In the blood type plan, there are highly beneficial foods and there are others to avoid. The highly beneficial are very good, even *medicinal* for your type. You may see some healthy foods on your avoid list simply because they don't agree with your type.

Health Coach Recommendations

Diverse proteins in the foods, called lectins, have agglutinating properties that affect the blood. Lectins can target an organ or bodily system, such as kidneys or digestive, and begin agglutination in that area. Therefore, adhering to our blood type diet prevents agglutination, promoting health and our ideal weight. While we can't choose our cards, knowing which foods to increase and which to decrease helps you play your winning hand.

Type "O" - strong, hunter, leader, self-reliant, goal-oriented

Strength	Weakness	Health Risk	Diet Profile	Weight Loss	Supple-ment	Exercise
strong immune system versatile adaptation to changes in diet and environ-ment strong nervous system tolerates chaos	no natural weak-nesses tendency toward auto-immune break-downs and rare viruses	type 1 diabetes chronic fatigue syndrome **<u>auto-immune disorders:</u>** Lou Gehrig's disease lupus multiple sclerosis	omnivore meat (no chicken) dairy[1] grains beans legumes vegetables fruit	**<u>reduce:</u>** corn lentils peanuts sesame seeds buckwheat wheat **<u>increase:</u>** greens eggs venison liver licorice tea	magne-sium licorice ginkgo lecithin	moderate physical, with mental balance **<u>such as:</u>** hiking biking tennis swimming

Type "O": American Indians 79%, Hispanic 57%, African Americans 49%, Caucasian Americans 45%, Western European 43%, Jewish 38%, Indians 37%, Japanese 30%, Chinese 30%, Korean 28%

Type "A" – cooperative, sensitive, orderly, settled, cultivator

Strength	Weakness	Health Risk	Diet Profile	Weight Loss	Supple-ment	Exercise
adapts well to changes in diet and enviro-ment little need for animal food immune system preserves and metabolizes nutrients more easily	sensitive digestive tract vulnerable immune system	heart disease cancer anemia liver and gallbladder disorders type 1 diabetes	classic vegan vegatarian vegetables tofu seafood grains beans legumes fruit	**reduce:** meat dairy kidney beans lima beans wheat **increase:** vegetables oil soy foods vegetables pineapple	vitamin B-12 for vegan type folic acid vitamin C vitamin E hawthorn echinacea	calming centering **exercises such as:** yoga tai chi

Western European 47%, Jewish 41%, Caucasian Americans 40%, Japanese 38%, Korean 32%, Hispanic 31%, African Americans 27%, Chinese 25%, Indians 22%, American Indians 16%

Type "B" – nomad, flexible, creative

Strength	Weakness	Health Risk	Diet Profile	Weight Loss	Supple-ment	Exercise
hardy digestive tract strong immune system natural defenses against infections efficent metabolism shorter small intestines less chance for cancer hardy digestive tract	low tolerance for new diets and new enviroments immune system can be over-active and attack itself	low thyroid inflammation arthritis blood-clotting disorders ulcers because they get overly acidic	red meat strong enzymes to digest meat high protein vegetables fruit	**<u>reduce:</u>** wheat/ corn[1] baked goods[2] kidney beans navey beans lentils brussel sprouts cauliflower mustard **<u>increase:</u>** kelp seafood liver red meat kale spinach broccoli	vitamin A vitamin K calcium iodine licorice kelp	intense physical exercise **<u>such as:</u>** running aerobics contact sports martial arts power yoga

Indians 33%, Korean 31%, Chinese 30%, Japanese 22%, African Americans 20%, Jewish 16%, Caucasian Americans 11%, Hispanic 10%, Western European 7%, American Indians 4%

Type AB – rare, enigma, mysterious, highly sensitive

Strength	**Weakness**	**Health Risk**	**Diet Profile**	**Weight Loss**	**Supple-ment**	**Exercise**
designed for modern life rugged immune system combined benefits of Type A and Type B	sensitive digestive tract tendency for over-tolerant immune system that allows for microbial invasion	heart disease cancer anemia	mixed diet in moderation meat seafood dairy tofu beans legumes grains vegetables fruit	**reduce:** red meat kidney beans lima beans seeds corn buckweat **increase:** tofu seafood good quality dairy greens kelp pineapple	vitamin C hawthorn echinacea valerian quercitin milk thistle	calming, centering exercises **such as:** yoga tai chi compined with moderate physical exercises **such as:** hiking cycling tennis

Japanese 10%, Korean 10%, Chinese 10%, Jewish 7%, Indians 7%, Caucasian Americans 4%, African Americans 4%, Western European 4%, Hispanic 2%, American Indians 1%

Recommended Readings:

Eat Right For (4) Your Type by James D'Adamo
Blood types Body types and You by Dr. Joseph Christiano

Spiritual Reflection of Blood

Only you shall not eat flesh with its life, that is, its blood (Gen. 9:4 NASB).

For the life of the body is in its blood (Lev. 17:11 NLT).

Blood is our life force. It provides nourishment by carrying oxygen and vital vitamins, minerals, and proteins throughout the body. The quality of our health is reflected in the quality of our blood. Pure, oxygenated blood is seen as a lighter, brighter color. Proper blood flow not only sustains life, but promotes healing.

So Jesus said to them, *"Truly, truly, I say to you, unless you eat the flesh of the Son of Man and drink His blood, you have no life in yourselves."* (John 6:53 NASB).

"I am the vine, you are the branches; he who abides in me and I in him, he bears much fruit, for apart from Me you can do nothing" (John 15:5 NASB).

Our Savior is our life force. As we receive and accept His sacrificial blood physically, symbolically, and spiritually in the sacrament of Holy Communion, we receive both spiritual wholeness and physical wholeness. As we cultivate our faith to receive both physical and spiritual wholeness, we receive the fullness of our salvation! The blood of the Lamb was spilled for complete body/soul/and spirit healing.

As a vine engrafted from the Divine Branch, His features emerge in us, even blossoming into all of our five senses. We become the sweet smell of Christ, the light of the world, the words of life, the sweet savior of Christ, and the healing touch of Christ to all whom we meet. Christ's Life makes our life flow with abundance. His blood not only sustains every aspect of our lives, but provides restorative power that leads to complete healing. Christ died once for all sin and His shed blood fully atoned for shortcomings and makes us children of the Most High. He is the vine fusing us with His continual presence, especially as we gather in fellowship, hearing his life-giving words and tasting the very nourishment that Jesus promised to give - his body, his blood, through the Holy Communion. Therefore, we are encouraged to gladly receive his precious gifts to us, his very life in body and spirit.

By Christ's blood, we have conquered sin, death, and the devil — therefore we are set free from fears, disease, and any weapons formed against us; by Christ's blood—we are set free!

"*They triumphed over him by the blood of the lamb* (Rev. 12:11).

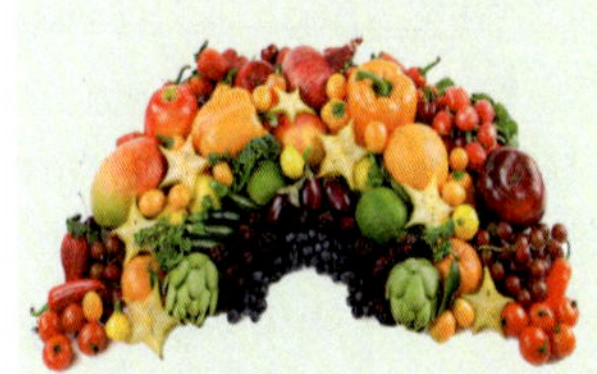

CHAPTER 7

The Science of Nutrition and Biblical Reflections

Then God said, "I give you every seed-bearing plant on the face of the whole earth and every tree that has fruit with seed in it. They will be yours for food (Gen. 1:29 NASB).

Everything that lives and moves about will be food for you. Just as I gave you the green plants, I now give you everything (Gen. 9:3 NASB).

When you choose from the cornucopia of foods that are in harmony with your genetic makeup, such as your blood and body type, you will naturally thrive. A generic diet, however, can be counterproductive to losing weight, and increasing energy. Every mammal should ideally select foods "according to its kind".

As we spotlight each category of the Food Pyramid, we'll see this *Gem of Genesis* from unique angles. Each food has special nutritional, medicinal, and energetics (qualities). When certain foods are combined together, they create a synergistic effect, which complements and multiplies their beneficial power. Add to this the color, shape, resemblance, and spiritual reflection, which all may radically change your relationship to food. In fact, it could become a creative art and a fun game – of *Clue.*

Have you ever watched a child play the game of *Clue*? See their eyes light up when they assemble the pieces and solve the mystery! Their faces burst with joy when they finally *get it*; and when they *get it*, they won't soon *forget* it.

Likewise, there are many clues mirrored in our food that serve to remind us of their amazing healing and healthful properties, which we'll explore throughout this section. May we be *wowed* as we uncover our Heavenly Father's clues for a lasting relationship with the food He provides.

Let's first look carefully at the food Pyramid. On the following pages is the previously used My Pyramid, familiar to many, and the Institute of Integrative Nutrition, (IIN), based on nutritional science. Here, we'll begin the game of *Clue*. On the following pages, carefully note the similarities and differences.

Compare MyPyramid to the following pyramid designed by the Institute for Integrative Nutrition (nutritional science). What do you see?

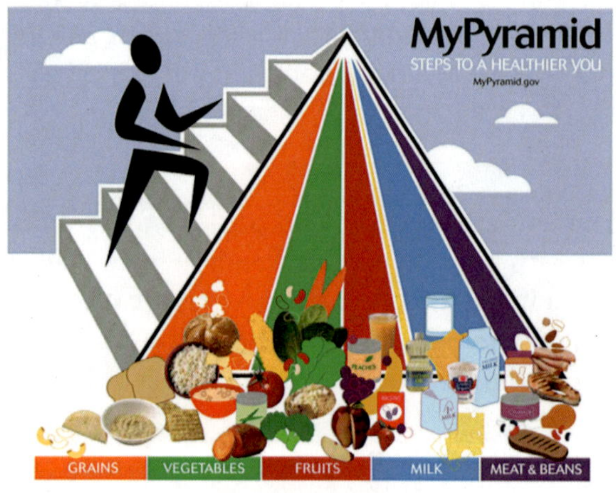

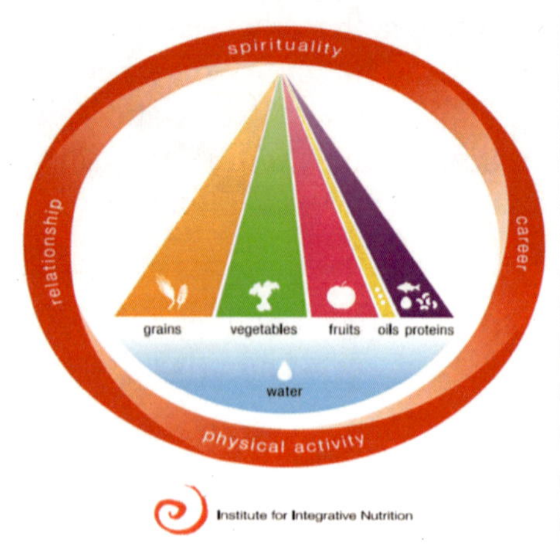

©2005 Integrative Nutrition Inc. (used with permission).

- MyPyramid begins with food categories but changes to food products, whereas they are consistently categories in the one below. Why might they change to products in the government Pyramid? What if they changed it to protein, rather than suggesting a product, such as milk or meat?
- In MyPyramid notice that the two products which are *proteins* consume about 35%, whereas in the one below, *protein* is about 25%. This is important for a balanced amount of *protien*, as we'll see later.
- Where is the vitally important category or product for *oils* in My Pyramid?
- The IIN Pyramid captures health in the big picture. Water is the foundation, the wellspring of nutrition that helps assimilate nutrition and remove toxins.
- In the IIN Pyramid, physical, or secondary food is surrounded by four soul nourishments, or primary foods: spirituality, relationships, career, and physical activity. These are like the four tires on your car. If one is out of alignment or flat, you're not cruising, no matter how many greens you eat. Thus, it encompasses the big picture of health.

These questions and comments are not intended to criticize but to raise awareness of nutrition as a precise science as we now enter the lush garden of Genesis, Glorious Greens under Vegetables. Though this is the second in the list, it is most crucial for our well being, and yet often the most neglected. Therefore, a double spotlight is displayed on these gems: one on greens, another on all other vegetables.

Glorious Greens

What makes greens so *glorious*?
Benefits of dark leafy greens:

- Purifies blood
- Prevents cancer

- Improves circulation
- Strengthens immunity
- Promotes digestion
- Increases energy
- Reduces depression
- Improves liver and kidney function
- Strengthens respiratory, prevents asthma and colds
- Creates emotional stability, a natural antidepressant
- Inspires creativity
- Nourishes bones with easily absorbable minerals

Suppose you could encapsulate all of those benefits into one pill; how much would it be worth? Yet, you can purchase a whole mess-a-greens for so little. The challenges for many of us is being unfamiliar with varieties of greens and preparing them appealingly. The solution: *Glorious Greens* (cookbook) and recommendations at the end of this chapter, but first, a fun game of *Clue*.

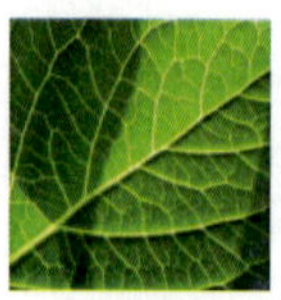

Clue 1. *Look at any edible leaf. What does its veiny structure resemble in the human body?*

Just as we are composed of tiny veins carrying oxygen and nutrition thoughout our whole bodily systems, so leafy greens have an intricate web that nourishes the whole plant. That's exactly what greens do for us, transporting nourishment into all of our organs and systems, even fotifying our mental and emotional state.

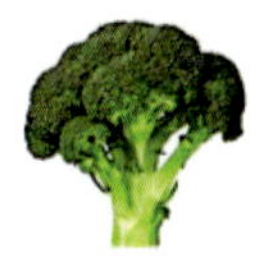

Clue 2. *Notice the growth pattern of greens. What does their upward and outward formation resemble in the human body?*

See how a *broccoli* looks like our bronchial system? Just as greens grow up and out, so our bronchial system goes up and out. Greens specifically *nourish our upper respiratory system.* They correlate with *our lungs,* which breathe up and out. In fact, they are the perfect complement to our lungs. Green plants take in carbon dioxide and give off oxygen, while our lungs take in oxygen and give off carbon dioxide. The energy of plants is mirrored and paralleled in our respiratory systems. Green plants are also high in chlorophyll, which helps supply our blood with oxygen. A primary function of greens is nourishing and supporting our respiratory system.

Clue 3. What does green mean?

Green is the color associated with spring, renewal, refreshment, and vital energy. It represents rejuvenation and balance; that's its effect on us. Isn't it amazing how the Lord placed Adam and Eve in the garden of greenery?

The dark green color reflects their mineral rich qualities, high in calcium, magnesium, iron, potassium, zinc and phosphorous. Greens are also vitamin rich, especially vitamins A, C, E, and K, and they're crammed with fiber and folic acid. Whenever possible, choose fresh, and better yet, organic.

The next clue is the growth pattern and colors of Root Vegetables.

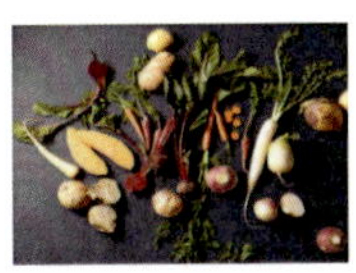

Notice the growth pattern of root vegetables. What does their downward formation resemble in the human body?

Root vegetables (those that grow underground) are the natural polarity to greens. Consider a carrot, having the opposite pattern of greens of downward and inward. As a root vegetable, it *absorbs and assimilates vital elements* from the soil for the entire plant. They correlate with the root of our bodies, our small intestinal. This is where we *mostly absorb and assimilate our food's nutrients.* Root vegetables' specific function is to nourish and support the lower intestine digestive system.

Growing downward, it is firmly *anchored* in the ground. The energy of a carrot then is *grounding and stability*. When do you need to feel more grounded? Perhaps when you're feeling emotionally and physically stressed from a lot of travel or activity. Root vegetables are natural comfort foods.

What are the color of most roots?

Most roots are warming colors, such as yellow, orange, and red. These stimulating and cleansing colors assist with many different types of digestive disorders. When certain roots are eaten together, they have a *synergestic* effect.

Synergy of vegetables

The concept of food synergy maintains that the key to good health is more than the individual healthy food you eat, but how you combine them, eating complementary foods that biochemically balance each other. Nature provides nutrition in concert, where the whole food is greater than the sum of its parts. Food Synergy is the right combinations that provide us with a full range of health benefits.

Certain foods and beverages interact with each other to give us extra disease protection and greater health. These vegetable combinations have a multiple of synergistic potential.

The term cruciferous refers to cool weather vegetables with four flowering petals, that resemble a *cross.* Indeed, these life-saving vegetables reflect this same spiritual quality. When combined, their synergetic effect is like the synergy of prayers – a multiplied impact. Veggies - Especially Dark Greens

Whether it's two vegetables high in fiber (eggplant and okra); the cruciferous veggies (like kale and broccoli) with their anticancer compounds; or a rich root mix (like carrots, sweet potatoes, and onions), the message is clear: the more the merrier, as they multiply their benefits, especially of their kind.

Tomatoes and broccoli - This combination is more effective at slowing prostate tumor growth than either is alone.

Cooked tomatoes with the peel on and healthy fats such as olive oil or avocado – Since most of the nutrition of tomatoes is in the skin, absorption of these key nutrients is much greater when the tomatoes are cooked in a healthy oil.

Cruciferous vegetables — Cruciferous vegetables are more active when combined. Researchers found that the two compounds were able to protect rats against liver cancer much better together, and they are known to activate important detoxification enzymes that help the body eliminate carcinogens before they harm our genes. Brussels sprouts and broccoli are ideal together with up to seven times greater benefits. Below are more of these anti-cancer superfoods.

Kale, Cauliflower, Brussels sprouts, Broccoli, Turnips, Collard Greens, and Mustard Greens

Vivacious vegetables

The cornucopia of vegetables provides an endless variety of flavors, aroma, and beauty. Their benefits are similar to those listed for greens, but each has their own energy and medicinal properties too. Many amazing clues are displayed in *God's Pharmacy.*

God's Pharmacy of Vegetables

Then God said, "Let the land burst forth with every sort of grass and seed-bearing plant. And let there be trees that grow seed-bearing fruit. The seeds will then produce the kinds of plants and trees from which they came. And so it was (Genesis 1:11 NASB).

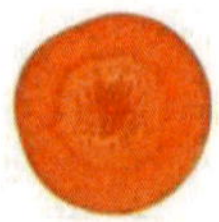

A sliced Carrot looks like the human eye. The pupil, iris, and radiating lines look just like the human eye...and YES science now shows that carrots greatly enhance blood flow to and function of the eyes.

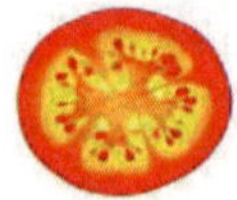

A Tomato has four chambers and is red. The heart is red and has four chambers. All of the research shows tomatoes are indeed pure heart and blood food.

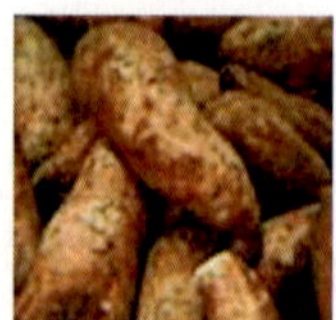

Sweet Potatoes - Sweet Potatoes look like the pancreas and help balance blood sugar levels.

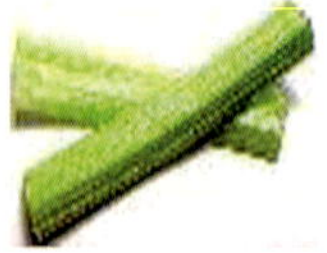

Celery, Bok Choy, Rhubarb, etc. look just like bones. These foods specifically target bone strength. Bones are 23% sodium and these foods are 23% sodium. If you don't have enough sodium in your diet, the body pulls it from the bones, making them weak. These foods replenish the skeletal needs of the body.

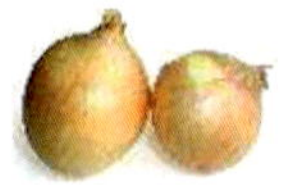

Onions look like body cells. Today's research shows that onions help clear waste materials from all of the body cells. They even produce tears which wash the epithelial layers of the eyes.

Below are the profiles of an array of this amazing superfood, greens, and preparation tips.

ARUGULA One of the most nutritious greens with more calcium than kale and collards and a peppery, flavor-enhancing quality as distinctive as its name. These spicy, pungent, warm nutty leaves can perk up a sandwich or salad, including pasta and potato salads, as they're part of the mustard family and a cruciferous.

BEET GREENS The edible and delicious tops are better sources of vitamin C, calcium, and iron than the beets themselves, though both are highly nutritious. Their dark wine color and complex flavor is mild, yet sweet. These greens are great in soups and with a variety of companions, such as dill, lemon, apples, oranges, and warm spices like cinnamon, nutmeg, cloves, and ginger.

BOK CHOY These delicately flavored leaves are loaded with Vitamin A and C, a cancer fighting cruciferous, and are so versatile, they're used in many Asian dishes. The high water content keeps the white crisp, yet succulent, while the leaves become tender, but still bright green. This delicate flavor may be your new crave.

BROCCOLI RABE and **BROCCOLI** The two are quite different. Broccoli Rabe, used in many Italian dishes, has a pungent, aggressive flavor with leaves and small florets, while broccoli is milder and bulkier. Broccoli Rabe adds zests to milder dishes, while broccoli gives crunch, substance, and its own unique taste.

CABBAGE This global green is enjoyed in a variety of ways around the world. It has been cultivated for 2,500 years and is great prepared almost every way: raw, steamed, boiled, stir-fried, added to soups and stews, and pickled. Its flavor can also be versatile, depending how it is cooked: sweet, sour, crisp, crunchy, or hearty. This cruciferous member stores well. Savoy cabbage (the crumpled leaves cabbage) has a more delicate, sweet taste; great for stuffing. Red cabbage is less sweet and tougher, but thin strips go nicely with salads.

CHARD Like spinach, it's one of the mildest tasting cooking greens: sweet, earthy, and succulent. It's also loaded with vitamins A and C, but is more durable than spinach. It, too, should be combined with other healthy oils to offset the oxalic acid, and goes well with olive oil and lemon juice. The two common forms are Swiss, with dark green glossy leaves, and Rhubarb, with red laced into the leaves.

CHINESE GREENS There's a great diversity among Chinese vegetables, offering various flavors and textures. Many have a delicate flavor and can be quickly stir fried for quick, healthy dishes. Some of these are Bok Choy, Napa, Pea Shoots, Chinese broccoli, Choy Sum, Tatsoi, Mustard Greens, Mizuna, and Water Spinach.

COLLARD GREENS A nutritional gem, though only well known in the South. Collard Greens are higher in nutritional value than broccoli, spinach, and mustard greens. The best way of cooking to preserve its nutrition is to quickly boil it for up to 8 to 10 minutes. Cooking greens quickly and lightly preserves nutrients, color, and taste. You can then sauté for added flavor. Collard greens are higher in nutritional value than broccoli, spinach, and mustard greens.

ENDIVE AND CHICORY These members of the thistle

family are often bitter herbs, usually a little thicker than other leaves. Most are high in Vitamin C and have a diuretic effect. They are medicinal in many countries. Some of these varieties are Escarole, Chicory, Frisee', Belgian Endive, and Radicchio.

GREEN BEANS AND PEAS These fibrous, fabulous greens are not so inspiring alone, but team them up with almost any combination of other vegetables, herbs, and main dishes, and you've got a winning combination.

KALE Known as "king of calcium," and a great crucifer, Kale is packed with fiber and Vitamins A, C, and 134 grams of calcium in one cup. Kale tastes good, too, especially quick-boiled, which retains its bright green color and brings out its tender sweetness. It can also be added to soup, stir-fried, or grilled. It's not recommended to be eaten raw unless it's the very tender garden baby kale.

LETTUCE AND SALAD GREENS Salads have come a long way, from a bland bowl of iceberg lettuce to colorful blends of greens, reds of many textures, flavors, and herbs. Such artistic mixes not only are appetizing, but offer nutritional variety. Salads can be a solo masterpiece or a lovely complement. The artistry of salad making is in blending salad greens from different groups. That is, blending crunchy, soft, spicy, sweet, mild, green, red, white, and herbs. Choose many varieties and create a different salad any time. Some of these varieties include Arugula, Batavian, Butterhead, Endive, Frisee', Loose-leaf, Mache, Mesclun, Miner's lettuce, Mizuna, Purslane, Red Orach, Radicchio, Romaine, and Watercress.

MUSTARD GREENS These spicy greens can be a challenge to make palatable. Served alone, it's like eating mustard alone. Yet it can be a nice enhancement in foods that need a little zip, such as beans, soups, and some root vegetables.

SPINACH This super food soars with antioxidant vitamins, A, C, and E, and is powered with many other nutrients, including more iron than most other greens. So it's no wonder that the man of Iron, Popeye, drank his spinach. Yet, it also contains more oxalic acid than most other greens, which binds with calcium and iron, making it difficult to assimilate these crucial minerals in the body. Healthy fats, however, eaten with spinach, counteract this effect, such as oils, cheese, or nuts/seeds. Therefore, it should be consumed with a healthy fat and in moderation. There are two common types of spinach: the flat, smooth type with a delicate flavor, which is generally preferred in salads and the savoy variety, with curly, crinkled leaves, with more substance, is better in cooked dishes.

TURNIP GREENS A close kin to mustard greens, a great source of calcium, iron, and other nutrients, but also one of the bitterest dark leafy greens. Quickly boiling in shallow water helps reduce bitterness.

WATERCRESS This perennial aquatic plant with small dark green leaves and hollow stems is truly a diamond in the stream. It's a cruciferous high in Vitamin A and B; is a good source of copper, iron, and magnesium; and has almost three times the calcium of spinach. It's peppery, spicy flavor, and dark green leaves can zip up many recipes with just a few. It complements salads, citrus, nuts, and tomatoes.

Watercress also has a rich history. When Hippocrates was searching for a hospital location, he insisted it be near a stream where watercress could grow. It was not only for the high nutritional value, but also for its energetic quality. As a water plant, it has a cleansing effect, especially medicinal for the kidney and bladder. This plant was used as an antibiotic, especially for kidney and bladder issues.

Enjoy a rich variety of greens and you will begin feeling renewal, refreshment, emotional stability, inspiring creativity, and vital energy!

Best Vegetables for each Blood Type

"O": artichoke, beet greens, broccoli, collard greens, escarole, ginger, kale, kelp, romaine, onion, okra, parsley, parsnip, peppers, sweet potato, pumpkin, spinach, Swiss chard.

"A": alfalfa sprouts, artichoke, beet greens, broccoli, carrot, celery, collard greens, escarole, garlic, ginger, kale, leek, romaine, mushroom, okra, onion, parsley, pumpkin, spinach, turnip.

"B": beet greens, broccoli, brussel sprouts, cabbage, carrot, cauliflower, collard greens, eggplant, ginger, kale, mushroom, mustard greens, parsley, parsnip, peppers, sweet potato, yam.

"AB": alfalfa sprouts, beet greens, broccoli, cauliflower, celery, collard greens, cucumber, eggplant, garlic, kale, mushrooms, mustard greens, parsley, sweet potato, parsnip, yam.

Health Coach Recommendations

- Be adventurous and try greens you've never tried before.
- Most greens need, a little company, to taste good. Some olive oil and herbs, garlic, sesame seeds, olives, or cranberries may be all it takes.
- Blend contrasts with color and tastes. Mix bibb lettuce with darker lettuce and pepper strips. Contrast parsley and dill with cabbage, spinach with mustard greens, etc. Blend sweet vegetables such as carrots, corn, squash, peppers, and tomatoes with rich green kale to become sweeter and more appealing.
- Nuts and seeds are a great match for greens. They are colorful, crunchy, tasty, and provide great protein and minerals for a complete balanced meal. Try pecans, walnuts, almond slices, sunflower seeds, pine nuts, and sesame seeds.
- Enjoy the foods you already eat by adding greens and other vegetables to pizza, omelets, soups, stews, pasta, and rice dishes.
- Use small amounts of healthy flavorful oils, such as sesame, avocado, or olive oil rather than saturating greens with bland processed fats and cheese.
- Tender greens like spinach, Swiss chard, and beet greens are best eaten in moderation because they are high in oxalic acid, which depletes calcium. Counter this effect by cooking

it with something rich like tofu, seeds, nuts, beans, butter, animal products, or oil. Eat moderately.

- Tougher greens with strong flavor, like kale, collards, turnip, and mustard greens are best cooked in shallow boiling water, becoming tender and less bitter. They can then be drained and sautéed.
- Cook greens in one to two cups of water, and save the water to add with soups, stews, smoothies, or cool and drink as a nutrient rich delicious "green cocktail."
- Boiling makes greens plump and relax, but quick boil to retain nutrients.
- Steaming makes greens more fibrous and tight, which is great for weight loss.
- Raw greens retain living enzymes, giving us more energy. They should be chewed well, and in moderation, as too much raw food may tax the digestive system.
- Fermenting greens, as in sauerkraut, is another healthy delicious alternative.

Recommended Reading:
Glorious Greens by Johnna Albi & Catherine Walthers

Eating greens and vegetables regularly rejuvenate and balance our lives in so many ways, providing us with endless benefits. Learning to prepare them in ways you enjoy is one of your greatest health investments. We now return to the Pyramid's first category, grains, great grains that sustain, but first, the spiritual reflection of greens.

Spiritual Reflection of Plants

He will be like a tree firmly planted by streams of water, which yields its fruit in its season and its leaf does not wither; and in whatever he does, he prospers (Psalm 1:3 NASB).

The Bible is filled with plant metaphors depicting a variety of spiritual qualities. Jesus frequently used plants in different contexts to express both the good and bad. Here our Lord meets us where we are: in the field, at the table, or simply observing the beauty of creation. Jesus uses plants as a universal language with global connections between plants and people. Knowing humanity's rich relationship with plants, his teachings weave in these analogies that help us harvest the rich kingdom of God.

Plants are not merely the backdrop of Jesus' stories – they are the main characters! Behold the lilies of the field…trusting for God's generous bounty; the tiny mustard seed is the seed of faith, and the word of God *springs forth*, germinating from small dried seeds and grows bountifully when cultivated. He summarized our relationship with him as, "I am the vine, you are the branches."

Trees and plants richly laced Jesus' ministry, symbolizing each aspect and transition. As a newborn, He was surrounded by *straw* in the manger, and with his entry into Jerusalem, he was surrounded by *royal palms*. He cursed the *fig tree*, and it dried up from its *roots*. He plucked Zacchaeus from the *sycamore fig tree*. He prayed in the garden of the Mount of *Olives*. He ate the last supper with *bitter herbs*. The soldiers stuck a sponge soaked in wine and held it up to Jesus on a branch of *hyssop* and raised it to His lips as He hung on a *tree*.

As our Lord *plucked* little Zacchaeus from the tree, who was *overtaxed* by sin, so he continues to *prune* the heavy burdens of sin and shame from our lives. Like plants, we are nurtured to flourish in every way. He removed the scorn and *thorns* of our sin when He wore the crown of **thorns* on his head.

In the Garden of Eden, the Lord God tells Adam that the earth will bring forth *thorns and thistles* because they ate the *forbidden fruit*. He bore this on the *tree* that our barren life could reap the bounty of eternity. In the fall, we were *thorns and thistles*; but in the resurrection to eternal life we are grafted as *branches, becoming one with* the beautiful life-sustaining V*ine,* that is

Christ our Lord, the Master *Vine Dresser*. Through Him, we are regenerated, blossoming in the fruit *of the Spirit*.

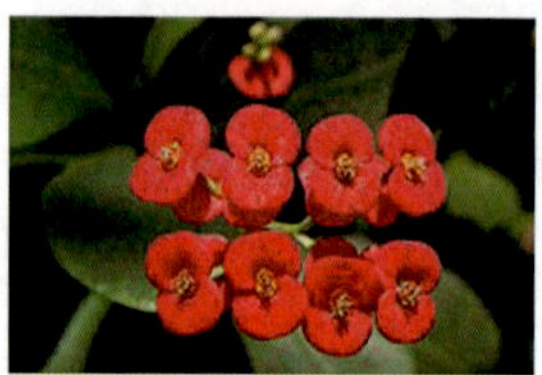

* Crown of Thorns, *Euphorbia milii*

Great Grains

No Grain, No Gain!
What is the great gain of the grain?

Benefits of Whole Grains:

Reduces most chronic disease:

- Heart disease by balancing cholesterol levels and blood pressure
- Cancer by cleansing and providing key nutrition
- Diabetes by regulating blood glucose
- Obesity, by fiber satisfying hunger, and cleansing

Whole grains are a great source of carbohydrate, which is an important source of energy for the body. Low-carb diets usually eliminate most whole grain foods and tend to be higher in fat. Unfortunately, the body can only store carbohydrate in limited amounts in the liver and muscles, and our diets must provide enough to meet our daily needs. Whole grains tend to be absorbed and digested more slowly, releasing energy slowly - helping you feel fuller for longer.

The fiber in whole grains is important for maintaining a healthy digestive system. Fiber helps speed the passage of waste material through the digestive system, giving potentially harmful substances less time to linger in the bowel and ensuring regular bowel movements.

Eating just three servings of wholegrain a day as part of a healthy diet and lifestyle, may help to reduce the risk of heart disease by up to 30%. Oats and barley contain a soluble fiber that has been shown to lower cholesterol and reduce heart disease.

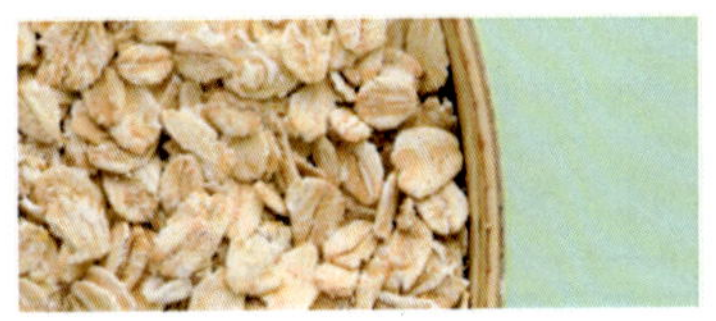

Clue 1 *Notice the tiny lines in whole grains.*

Compare whole grain oats with highly processed oats, or natural brown rice with white rice. When these lines were *stripped* (processed), what else was *stripped*? *About 25% of a grain's protein and at least seventeen key nutrients are lost in processing.*

What are Whole Grains?

A grain is considered whole when all three parts – *the bran, germ, and endosperm* – are present. Whole grains are key nutrients, like fruits and vegetables. In fact, whole grains are a good source of B vitamins, Vitamin E, magnesium, iron, and fiber, as well as other valuable antioxidants not found in some fruits and vegetables. Most of the antioxidants and vitamins are found in the germ and the bran of a grain.

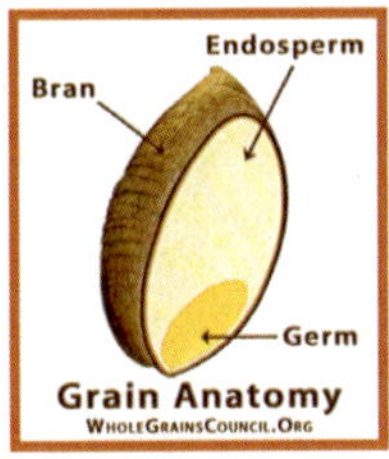

The Bran

The bran is the multi-layered outer skin of the kernel that protects it from pests and disease. It contains important antioxidants, B vitamins, and fiber.

The Germ

The germ is the embryo which can sprout into a new plant. It contains many B vitamins, some protein, minerals, and healthy fats.

The Endosperm

The endosperm provides essential energy to the young plant so it can send roots down for water and nutrients and send sprouts up for sunlight's photosynthesizing power. It contains proteins and small amounts of vitamins and minerals.

Whole grains contain all three parts of the kernel. Refining normally removes the bran and the germ, leaving only the endosperm. *Without the bran and germ, about 25% of a grain's protein is lost and at least seventeen key nutrients.* Processors add back some vitamins and minerals to enrich refined grains to try to compensate for what was lost. This manmade fortifying, however, is not the same nutritionally as it was.

Whole grains may be eaten whole, cracked, split, or ground. They can be milled into flour or used to make bread, pasta, or cereal. A "whole grain" product is required to have virtually the same proportions of bran, germ, and endosperm as the harvested kernel does before it is processed.

Clue 3. Look for the whole grain stamp.

This is actually a manmade clue, but a quick reference that makes shopping a little easier.

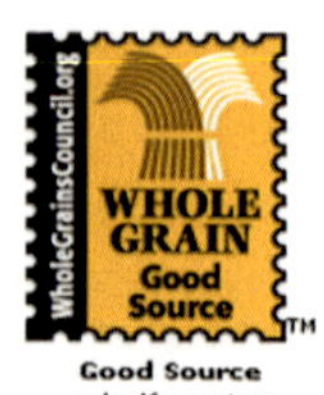

Good Source
a half serving
of whole grain

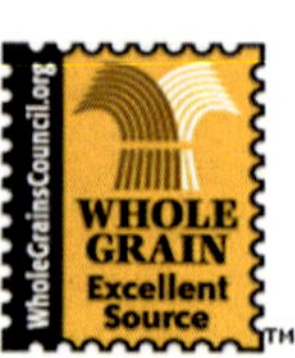

Excellent Source
a full serving
of whole grain

This stamp is on most, but may not be on all, whole grains. When determining if a product contains whole grain or not, look for the word "whole" in the ingredient list. Also, look for the Whole Grain Stamp. A "good source" stamp contains at least a half serving of whole grains, and an "excellent source" contains at least one serving of whole grains.

Foods labeled with the words "multi-grain," "stone-ground," "100% wheat," "cracked wheat," "seven-grain," or "bran" are not necessarily whole-grain products. Brown does not necessary mean whole wheat or whole grain because some breads have brown coloring added. Again, look for the words "whole grain."

Clue 2. See the natural earthy colors of whole grains.

Most grains are some shade of brown. Brown is a rich, earthy color, but is so bland that it needs a complimentary color to enhance it. Just a touch of gold or yellow is all that's needed to *lighten up* brown. Likewise, the taste of most grain is like this: earthy but bland, and needs the touch of condiments, spices, fruit, etc. to bring it to life. This is often the greatest obstacle, finding those golden touches that bring zest or tang to the grain. For this, see the whole grain cookbooks at the end of this chapter. The bright side of the bland side is *unlimited versatility.*

Go with the Grain

Every culture is *in-grained* with their traditional grains: India and Asia, rice; Americas, corn; Africa, sorghum; Middle East, wheat, tabouli, and coucous; Scotland, oats; Russia, buckwheat or kasha; and Europe, millet, wheat, rice, corn (producing their staple healthy beverage - *beer*). Whole grains are an excellent source of nutrition, which contain essential enzymes, iron, fiber, and many minerals and vitamins. Weight can be easily managed by consuming the ideal grains for your blood type.

Here is the profile of some main grains.

Brown Rice

- Generates energy
- Promotes good digestion
- Quenches thirst
- Alleviates diarrhea caused by spleen-pancreas deficiency
- Relieves mental depression

The many varieties of rice allows a perfect texture and flavor for each dish. Long grain rice is light and fluffy, while short grains are a bit sticky. Some rices are aromatic and delicious, like Jasmine and Basmati, because of their delicate or nutty aroma and flavor.

Brown rice has all bran layers intact and all of its naturally present nutrients. Brown rice has the highest amount of B vitamins out of all grains. Additionally, it contains iron, vitamin E, amino acids, and linoleic acid, and is high in fiber. Brown rice and other grains should be soaked to produce beneficial enzymes, increase availability of nutrients, and reduce phytic acid which prevents proper mineral absorption.

Oats

- Highest fiber grain
- May lower blood pressure
- Reduces risk of coronary artery disease
- Lowers risk of colorectal cancer

Unlimited versatility in one little word –OATS! Oats are not just for milk and cookies. Oats make satifying soups, stews, chili, tacos, meatloaf, pies, pizza crust, biscuits, pancakes, and an amazon of desserts! (See Oatrageous Oatmeals.)

Oats are unique in the way they are sliced or diced, which actually changes their flavor. For instance, the coarser steel-cut have a nuttier, crunchier flavor, while rolled oats have a mild, creamy texture. Oat flour is also an excellent whole grain option for baking since it's gluten-free and lighter and fluffier than whole wheat flour.

Quinoa

- A complete protein containing all eight amino acids
- High in B vitamins, iron, zinc, potassium, calcium, and vitamin E
- Gluten-free; easy to digest
- Ideal food for endurance
- Strengthens the kidneys, heart, and lungs

Quinoa (pronounced keen-wah) is a nutritional powerhouse with the highest nutritional profile. It is an extremely high-energy grain which has been grown and consumed for about 8,000 years on the high plains of the Andes Mountains in South America.

Quinoa cooks quickly. As it cooks, the outer germ surrounding the seed breaks open to form a crunchy coil while the inner grain becomes soft, translucent, and delicious.

Wheat

- Nutrient dense grain
- Wide spectrum of vitamins and minerals
- Reduces risk of heart disease
- Lessens chronic inflammation

Whole wheat is a great way to make pastas, breads, and cookies into a healthy treat that still maintains a soft texture and stability.

Alternately, those who are wheat intolerant can use other whole grains. If you think you may have an intolerance or allergy, it is important to be properly diagnosed. Gluten-free grains include rice, corn, buckwheat, millet, and quinoa, and pure, uncontaminated oats.

Since whole grains are so crucial in protecting our health, wouldn't it be great to make a grain bank from which you could quickly withdraw? That's exactly what Lorna Sass suggests in *Whole Grains Every Day Every Way.* This encourages healthy, convenient meal preparation. Uncooked grains can be preserved by being placed in sealed containers and stored in a cool dry place, or cooked grains can be refrigerated or put in freezer, for lasting quality.

Best Grains for each Blood Type

"O": oats, quinoa, buckwheat/kasha, rice, rye, spelt, sprouted grain bread (avoid wheat)

"A": buckwheat/kasha, oats, rye, barley, bulgur, coucous, rice, spelt, sprouted grain bread

"B": millet, oats, rice, spelt, barley, quinoa

"AB": oats, rice, rye, spelt, bulgur, couscous, quinoa

Health Coach Recommendations

- Replace white bread with whole grain bread.
- Enjoy whole grain breakfast cereal in the morning.
- Try oat or whole wheat flour in cookies, muffins, quick breads, and pancakes.
- Add brown rice, wild rice, or barley in soups.
- Snack on popcorn instead of chips on movie nights.
- Store up your grains (like Joseph).

The Synergy of Whole Grains

Whole grains are naturally low in fat and cholesterol-free, containing protein and loads of fiber, minerals, vitamins, and antioxidants. Whole grains are a synergistic explosion by itself, providing so many health benefits, including protection from heart disease, stroke, diabetes, obesity, and cancer.

Recommended Reading:

Whole Grains Every Day Every Way by Lorna Sass
Oatrageous Oatmeals by Kathy Hester
The New Whole Grains Cookbook by Robin Asbell

Spiritual Reflection of Grains

Grain Offering

In the Old Testament, there were two primary types of sacrifices made to the Lord: the animal sacrifice and the grain offering. In modern time, the first would be similar to tithing, honoring God with our first fruits, demonstrating our trust in God as our sole provider. The second would parallel giving of ourselves in servitude.

The grain offering was unique because the faithful people of God participated in the creation of their offering by their agricultural practice, and then grinding into flour and mixing with oil. In this way, they imparted their energy, focus, and skills into the offering, becoming a part of this holy sacrifice. Likewise, when we serve or volunteer, we are demonstrating the spirit of the grain offering.

When anyone brings a grain offering as an offering to the LORD, his offering shall be of fine flour. He shall pour oil on it and put frankincense on it (Lev. 2:1 ESV).

Notice the first requirement is that the offering shall be made of fine flour. It must be the finest quality. He shall pour oil on it. Oil is penetrating and we are anointed with the penetrating oil of the Holy Spirit. This allows our imperfect humanity to present a perfect sacrifice of which we are incapable of without the

Holy Spirit. When our offering is made with the pure love of God, it becomes a sweet smelling sacrifice, like the sweet aroma of frankincense.

No grain offering, which you bring to the Lord, shall be made with leaven, for you shall not offer up in smoke any leaven or any honey as an offering by fire to the Lord (Lev. 2:11 NASB).

Leaven symbolized impurity. In biblical times, it referred to physical impurity, and in our time, it can imply purity of thought, heart, and motive. We present a pure offering with the help of the Holy Spirit, who searches the depths of the heart, and the word of God, that purifies us seven times.

In our fast paced, competitive, multi-tasking world, we must consciously focus and meditate on our perfect *grain sacrifices*. It may be coordinating a program, trimming bushes, or actually preparing grains to make cookies or bread. It could be reaching out to help someone stand tall, writing an encouraging note, or simply embracing someone.

Whatever your offering may be, let it be the best, and the best of you! Seek to understand how His anointing will carve new paths that you never imagined and loosen rusted strongholds, with like lubricating oil! Smile, knowing that your wholehearted love emanates as a pleasing aroma; pray, realizing that prayer truly moves mountains; and think on those things that are lovely and of good report. May he *grind* our shortcomings and *blend* us with His Holy Spirit, that we will *rise* to be a most delectable aroma to the Lord.

Fantastic Fruits

What is the *fountain of youth*? It is a *fountain* of fruit with streams of apples, oranges, peaches, and pears cascading through bountiful trees. It is a vinyard of grapes, strawberries, and blueberries with rejuvenating antioxidants streaming right into our cells.

Benefits of Fruits:

- Cleanses Internally (at cellular level)
- Cleanses Externally (supple skin texture and vibrant glow)
- Bursting with essential minerals and vitamins that help fend off disease
- Improves health, weight, regulates blood circulation and digestion
- Full of antioxidants, preventing cellular damage

Clue 1. *How does the oxidation of an apple mirror our internal oxidation process?*

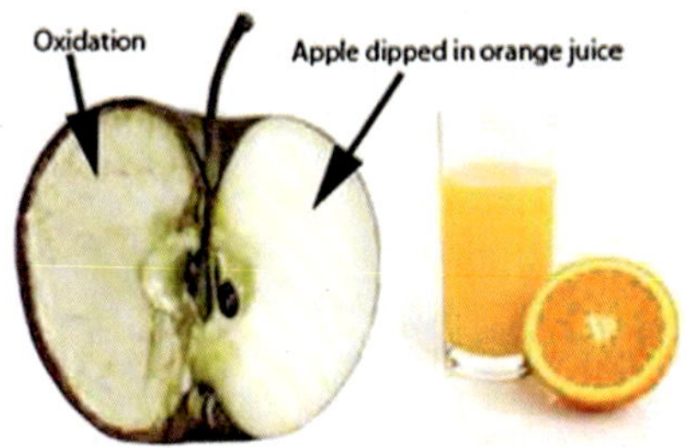

What makes fruits so fantastic is that they help prevent oxidation in our cells. Oxidation is like rusting on the inside. Yet the synergy of fruits full of antioxidants, combined with rich minerals and vitamins, prolong the natural aging process of wrinkling skin, hair loss, memory loss, and macular degeneration. Like citrus fruits, such as lemons and oranges, freshen and renew apples, so fantastic fruits rejuvenate our cells, organs, and tissues.

Clue 2. *What is the significance of fruit colors?*

Each color of fruits has specific benefits that correlate with the colors in the human body.

Red and Purple fruits protect against *heart* disease, *blood* clots, cancer, Alzheimer's disease, and improve *blood* circulation.

Yellow, Orange, and Green fruits boost the immune system and support eye and *skin* health.

White fruits help lower cholesterol, regulate blood pressure, and prevent cancer (*white* blood cells balanced).

See how the colors, textures, and shapes of common fruits reveal clues to their benefits.

Strawberries

- Red color, heart-shape that fight diseases which help lower risk of heart attack
- Great fiber, prevent constipation, lowers glucose levels and blood cholesterol
- Powerful antioxidant, prevents free radicals and diseases
- Build strong bones
- Protects against Alzheimer's disease and cancer
- Promote good function of metabolism

Apples

- Prevent osteoporosis, increase bone density, and strengthen bones
- Reduce asthma
- Protect brain cells from damage that may lead to Alzheimer's disease
- Reduce cholesterol
- Remove toxic substances, for intestinal health by increasing good bacteria
- Reduce the risk of kidney disease and kidney stones

Bananas

- Activate the mind and memory, improve mental alertness
- Provide the body with energy and protein
- Natural remedy for Anemia because they contain iron
- Regulates mood and calm the brain
- Replenish moisture to skin, and shine to hair
- Prevent hypertension

Oranges (and orange fruit)

- Regulate the digestive system, prevent constipation, and remove toxins from colon
- Stabilize blood sugar levels
- Boost the immune system and fight infections
- Promote healthy bones and teeth
- Maintain body fluids, regulate blood pressure, and prevent muscle cramps
- Protect the skin, accelerate wound healing, keep skin soft, and reduce signs of aging

Blueberries

- Top antioxidant boosting immunity and preventing illness
- Reduce body fat
- Decrease risk of cardiovascular disease
- Promote healthy urinary tracts
- Support brain health
- Improve digestion and prevent constipation

Grapes

- Accelerate weight loss
- Protect the heart and lower blood pressure
- Improve mental processes and responses
- Reduce inflammation
- Support muscle recovery
- Activate the longevity gene

Pineapples

- Help digestion
- Promote weight loss
- Are anti-inflammatory
- Prevent hypertension
- Promote eye health, preventing macular degeneration
- Maintain clear and glowing skin

Cherries

- Potent cancer prevention
- Promote better sleep

- Improve eyesight
- Help with weight loss
- Boost memory function
- Relieve arthritis

Watermelons

- Keep your body hydrated with electrolytes
- Cleanse kidneys and remove toxins
- Promote weight loss
- Increase brain function and reduce stress
- Protect skin damage and rejuvenate skin
- Regulates heart rate and blood pressure

Lemons

- Relieve digestive issues
- Diminish aging symptoms in skin
- Reduce throat and repiratory problems
- Accelerate weight loss
- Decrease gum and teeth infections
- Stabalize blood pressure and reduce stress

Clue 3. *Why do citrus and berries sprout in the spring and apples fall in the fall?*

Fruit helps prevent disease, is naturally cleansing, and even helps us transition into the next season. They help regulate all of our bodily systems, such as digestive, circulatory, and even our temperature.

Have you ever wondered why certain fruits grow at particular seasons? Consider how their qualities affect our bodies and marvel at our Creator's perfect seasonal timing.

In the late winter/early spring, we have citrus fruits and some berries. They are especially cleansing, washing us from winter accumulation and spring pollen, as do heavy spring rains wash the earth of its debris. They boost our immunity at a time when we may be weakened from lack of sunlight during the winter. They also replenish moisture in our skin from winter dehydration.

Then summer brings an array of melons and fibrous fruits. Watermelon contains electrolytes to maintain hydration and lycopene, a natural UV skin protection. Cantaloupe and honeydew also have ultra-cooling effects on the body. High fiber fruits, such as peaches, apricots, and plums, give sustained energy to carry us through the long, hot summer days.

After the summer, in the fall, apples ripen. Apples purge the summer heat from our bodies to gradually prepare us for winter. Apples remove toxins that may have become stagnant in our bodies through the summer and help regulate our digestive system, cleansing our colon. They also clear our upper respiratory after summer humidity and prepare us to breathe easier for the harsh winter weather.

In the late fall, we harvest the nutrient packed, super food, pumpkin. At this time, we become more sedentary and may easily put on weight. But pumpkin comes to our rescue; it's extremely high in fiber and helps us feel fuller longer and eat less. Also, its free radical neutralizing powers helps condition our skin for the coming dry winter. It boosts our immunity for the winter and even sharpens our eyesight! What a great time to see clearly, when nature camouflages with lovely fall and winter scenery. What's more, pumpkin seeds increase serotonin production, the hormone that enhances good moods. What a great antidote to winter the blues!

You need not remember all of these qualities; just remember to eat an abundance of the fruit when they are provided in each season.

Best Fruits for each Blood Type

"O": banana, blueberry, cherry, fig, guava, mango, plum, and prune

"A": apricot, all edible berries, fig, grapefruit, lemon, lime, pineapple, plum, and prune

"B": banana, cranberry, grape, papaya, pineapple, plum, and watermelon

"AB": cherry, cranberry, fig, grape, grapefruit, kiwi, lemon, pineapple, plum, and watermelon

Health Coach Recommendations

- Add cleansing fruit (citrus slices or berries) to your drinking water
- Consume plenty of the fruit that is medicinal for your conditions
- Enjoy plenty of the fruit that is in season to reap seasonal benefits
- Add fruit to yogurt, smoothies, parfaits, salads, and main dishes.
- Choose fresh (organic preferably) or frozen fruit
- Choose pure, fresh juice containing natural fiber and no added sugar
- Eat fruit consistently for pure skin, internal cleansing, and youthful glow
- Ward off disease and slow the aging process with daily fruits

Recommended Reading:

Ripe, A Fresh Colorful Approach to Fruits and Vegetables
by Cheryl Sternman Rule

Spiritual Reflection of Fruit

But the fruit of the Spirit is love, joy, peace, forbearance, kindness, goodness, faithfulness, gentleness, and self-control (Gal: 5:22).

God implores us to enter into a true sanctification process with Him so that He can cultivate us into the fully mature, richly ripened expression of His image. As we flourish in these nine fruits of the Spirit, we become the sweetest aroma to the world.

Like the cluster of grapes naturally suckle life as they ripen on the vine, so we draw these divine attributes into the core of our personalities. Similarly, as infants suckle from their mothers and milk begins to flow, the infant must initiate the flow. So, too, must we draw from the living water – Jesus, asking the Holy Spirit to fill us with these nine divine qualities.

LOVE is the greatest virtue that is placed above all else, even above faith and charity. Every benevolent act filters through the gold standard of love.

"If I speak in the tongues of men or of angels, but do not have love, I am only a resounding gong or a clanging cymbal. If I have the gift of prophecy and can fathom all mysteries and all knowledge, and if I have a faith that can move mountains, but do not have love, I am nothing. If I give all I possess to the poor and give over my body to hardship that I may boast, but do not have love, I gain nothing.

Love is patient, love is kind. It does not envy, it does not boast, it is not proud. It does not dishonor others, it is not self-seeking, it is not easily angered, it keeps no record of wrongs. Love does not delight in evil but rejoices with the truth. It always protects, always trusts, always hopes, always perseveres. Love never fails... (I Cor. 13: 1-8).

As these qualities emerge into rich hues, our love for God, ourselves, others, and even our enemies blossoms into greater dimensions and intensity. We pray for our enemy rather than despise him, we reach out to our brethren rather than pass them by, we esteem ourselves as royalty, and we cannot help but worship our loving God.

JOY Pressure and challenges can pierce our balloon of joy, leaving us spiraling to the ground, yet God inflates us with a fresh breath of His divine joy, restoring us with an even deeper joy.

The joy of The Lord is our strength (Neh. 8:10). This was Jesus' strength during His excruciating sacrifice. *For the joy set before him he endured the cross…* (Heb. 12:2).

The joy of The Lord can infuse us with His mighty power during tough times, especially as we praise and worship Him during challenges. It is His joy that hydrates our soul, even when ours is all dried up. Joy is gladness of heart, a deep inner rejoicing, and a great delight that re-inflates our spirit.

PEACE It's easy to become shaken and rattled from the daily stressors of relationships and work to extreme health crisis and trauma. Yet, even during these circumstances, our Lord calms the storm inside of us. The peace of The Lord can keep us emotionally stable, even during a crisis.

Therefore we will not fear, though the earth do change, and though the mountains be shaken into the heart of the seas… (Psalm 46:2 ASV).

This is the peace that surpasses human understanding, filling us with a sense of well-being, by His divine presence. "Even though You walk through the shadow of Darkness, you Shall not fear—for Your God shall lead you beside the still waters and provide a banquet, even in the midst of your trials. When we train our spirit to tread through turbulent waters, The Lord can direct us into a new *current*, a solution, or a greater perception that comes from His divine wisdom."

LONGSUFFERING is a long word that stretches our patience while we wait for the Lord to brew the good things He has in store for us, or slowly churn hearts and circumstances. We're acclimatized to our fast paced world where we expect expedient answers or changes. Yet, when we reflect on what God has done, we know He is continuing to do good work in us behind the scenes. We wait upon The Lord and rewind to His time zone, where *One thousand years in your sight are but a single day* (Psalm 90:4 ISV).

KINDNESS Our *impatience* can cause us to lose our sense of *kindness* and respect. Yet, a simple kind word or action can change someone's day, even their life! Our kindness is reflected in the quality of our love. It is love in action demonstrated as hospitality, service, friendship, benevolence, and graciousness. It is the hands and heart of Jesus reaching out in a special way, which in turn reaches back and touches us. *Kindness is the harvest of love.*

GOODNESS It is the goodness of God that brings a man to repentance and salvation. This powerful, magnetic energy draws people to God through the believer. Many have come to know The Lord due to the charisma of love and goodness. We are to let our light shine without hesitation. When people sense this genuine godly goodness, they often feel secure and begin to open to receive the fullness of the Lord's goodness. Goodness is a kind heart in action, generosity, and the full expression of God.

FAITHFULNESS The scriptures portray faith as being steadfast in the midst of turbulent waves. In this day of raging waters in families, friendships, and career, we need The Lord to help us to remain steadfast in what He has prepared for us. He gives us the grace to continue in His plan for our lives in some amazing way. Faithfulness is the unwavering loyalty to God that makes us steadfast in other relationships and our own aspirations.

GENTLENESS Jesus was our perfect role model. He knew when to respond with gentleness that transformed a sinner's life, and he knew when to respond sternly to his adversaries. Likewise, the Holy Spirit guides us to reach forth with a gentle word or touch, or a firm approach, when appropriate.

Parents can lose this balance when disciplining children. Sometimes, tough love is needed, but other times, gentleness is the best approach for healthy development. Gentleness is the characteristic of one who rules *his own spirit* well. Gentleness might be perceived as weak or feminine; yet it flowed through Jesus, the most powerful, strongest man ever.

SELF-CONTROL is the precursor to gentleness, and in fact, to all of the fruit of the Spirit. Our materialistic world is designed to prey on our impulsive sin nature. Yet, the spirit of the Lord allows us to launch out into the deep where true freedom and real wealth enrich our lives.

Without self-control, we are imprisoned by a judgmental, critical, unforgiving spirit, or enslaved to addictions and attachments. Ironically, those who fail to control themselves often try to control everyone else. Temperance allows us to be *in this world*, but not *of this world*.

As you see, the nine fruits of the Spirit work harmoniously together in supporting the development of our inner man. We become this voluptuous fruit as we devote our attention, words, and actions to these traits.

The fruit of the Spirit is spiritually cleansing from the *inside out*, washing us from all negative emotions and motives. It is our spiritual antioxidant, *anti-rusting* quality, preserving our fresh aroma. It sanctifies or sets us apart from the world "where rust and moths corrupt."

The Fruit of the Spirit is *from* the Spirit. Only by prayer and abiding in God's word can your relationship remain fertile, that you harvest the Fruit of the Spirit in your life.

The next in the Pyramid's lineup is a category that not too long ago was considered an unhealthy food, but now we understand its crucial role in our well-being: oils and fats.

Fabulous Fats

A few decades ago, fats were not so fabulous. In fact, we squeezed every drop of oil from our diet, hoping to lose fat. Ironically, we *increased* in fat! We were on the low-fat craze and all fats were considered bad. Now we understand the nutritional value of fats, and that healthy fats actually help maintain a lean body. So what have we learned about fats and oils - the good, bad, and ugly? Let's start with ugly and work our way to good.

Processed Trans-fat (trans-fatty acids) – now that's downright ugly! It raises your LDL ("bad") cholesterol and lowers your HDL ("good") cholesterol, increasing your risk of many health risks, such as heart disease. Most trans-fat is formed through an industrial process that adds hydrogen to vegetable oil, causing the oil to become solid at room temperature, allowing a longer shelf life.

Trans fat, known as *partially hydrogenated oil*, is found in a variety of food products, including cakes, cookies, pie crusts, crackers, ready-made frosting, chips, microwave popcorn, deep fried foods, refrigerated dough products, creamers, and margarines. Avoid all foods and liquids with hydrogenated oils, or trans-fat, and these highly processed oils.

Margarine, made of synthetic trans-fat (as opposed to the naturally occurring trans-fats found in some meat and dairy products) is one of the worst fats. These trans-fat-free margarines are replaced with *another* chemically constructed fat that may increase blood sugar and insulin resistance, and still lowers good and increases bad cholesterol, increasing your risk of heart disease, diabetes, and weight gain!

Soybean oil, also known as vegetable oil, is like margarine. It's high in omega-6 fatty acid, but we need a balance of omega-6 and omega-3 fatty acids for optimal health. This imbalance contributes to obesity and other serious health issues. It's unstable and goes rancid quickly. Rancid oils form free radicals that can lead to cancer, accelerated aging, and other diseases. When it's heated, it goes rancid even faster. Some soybean oils may be rancid before you even begin cooking due to heat and light exposure during storage and transport. Most soybeans are now genetically modified, which is linked to fertility problems, allergies, etc.

Corn oil is like soybean oil, with a significant imbalance of far more omega-6 fats than omega-3 fats. Corn oil goes rancid fairly quickly on the shelf and even faster in the frying pan.

Canola oil is typically highly processed, contains trans-fats, and is easily damaged by heat.

Now see the great benefits of *good fats.*

- Improve body composition
- Increase muscle mass, decrease body fat
- Support reproductive health
- Boost brain function and mood
- Strengthen bones
- Enhance heart health, improve cholesterol ratio
- Provide better skin and eye health
- Decrease the pain and stiffness of arthritis

Clue 1: *Compare the rich color, scent, taste and texture of natural oils with processed.*

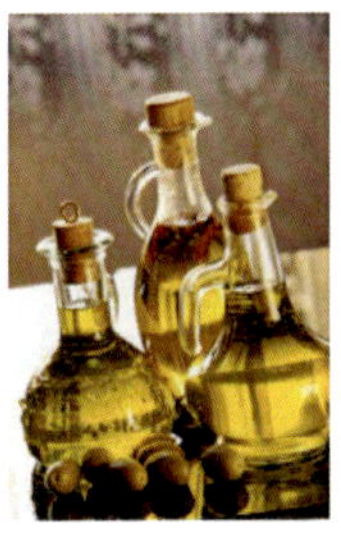

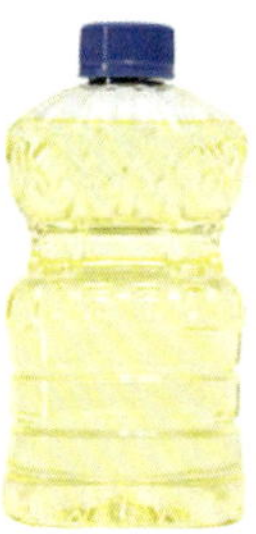

The full bodied color and aroma reflect the rich minerals and vitamins which emanate from the plant from which the oil was derived. Highly processed oils have been stripped of these elements and have been replaced with the health risks stated earlier.

Clue 2: *How does the lubricating quality of oil impact our body?*

A deficiency in healthy fats can lead to dry skin and eyes and stiff joints. An adequate level of omega-3s and a variety of saturated fats helps the body's lubricating system operate efficiently. Have you checked *your* oil lately? If you're starting to feel like the *tin man,* check out these fabulous fats.

Monounsaturated fats, liquid at room temperature, and solid when they are chilled, are a healthy alternative to the trans-fats, refined polyunsaturated, saturated fats in most processed foods. They raise good cholesterol and lower the bad. Some great sources are in unprocessed plant oils, avocados, and nuts.

OLIVE OIL is a heart healthy synergy combining both a high content of monounsaturated fatty acids and a high antioxidant level.

The purer forms contain higher nutritional value:

- **Extra virgin** is considered the best, least processed, comprised of oil from the first pressing. It is extracted using a cold press without heat or chemicals, retaining a pure flavor, and higher levels of antioxidants, particularly vitamin E, as it's less processed.
- **Virgin** is from the second pressing.
- **Pure** undergoes some processing, such as filtering and refining, made by adding a little extra virgin olive oil to refined oil, a lower grade labeled as just "olive oil."
- **Light** undergoes considerable processing for a mild olive flavor and may be mixed with other vegetable oils.

Olive oil has a low heat tolerance and shouldn't be cooked at a high temperature. Use to lightly sauté, drizzle on salads, vegetables, grains, meats, etc.

Olive oil is very well tolerated by the stomach and helps prevent colon cancer, ulcers, and gastritis. It activates the secretion of bile and pancreatic hormones much more naturally than prescribed drugs. Consequently, it lowers the incidence of gallstone formation.

GRAPESEED OIL is another heart healthy champion, preventing high blood pressure and atherosclerosis, reducing cholesterol, and supporting the circulatory system for healthy blood vessels. Other benefits include the following:

- High in vitamin E, it makes a great remedy for stretch marks and can be used on delicate areas of the face, such as under the eyes, spreading well on the skin.
- Used to treat eczema and dry skin. The emollient effect lubricates the skin and is used by massage therapists.
- Can reduce complications from diabetes when added to the diet.

Grapeseed oil is pressed from the seeds of grapes used in wine-making. It is naturally high in vitamin E, omega-3 fatty acids, omega-6 fatty acids, and contains traces of very powerful anti-oxidants.

Grapeseed oil has a high heat tolerance (how much it can be heated before burning), that allows a higher smoke point; it doesn't break down like other oils and is nutritionally more stable. This property, combined with its neutral flavor, makes it perfect for frying and sautéing. It can be reused, retaining pleasant flavors and odors. Its mild neutral flavor allows the other flavors of the food to shine through. Like Olive oil, it can be blended with many foods.

AVOCADO OIL is derived from the avocado fruit, boasting many healthy properties. Avocado oil is high in vitamin E and unsaturated fats and contains more protein than any other fruit and more potassium than a banana. Avocado oil (and avocados) offers a variety of nutritional and medicinal benefits.

- Nutrient absorption of a salad with avocado is as much as 15 times greater
- Lowers Blood Pressure in response to hormones that regulate blood pressure
- Stimulates cartilage growth and repair for treating knee and hip osteoarthritis

- Reduces bone erosion associated with periodontal disease
- Improves psoriasis by using a blend of vitamin B12 and avocado oil cream
- Decreases hair loss and dandruff and is easily absorbed into the scalp and skin
- Acts as a deep skin moisturizer when applied directly on skin or in a soothing bath

The rich buttery texture of avocado oil brings a royal enhancement to many dishes. It has a heat tolerance exceeding 500 degrees, the highest smoke point of any natural oil, allowing cooking versatility such as stir-frying, searing, broiling, and frying. It can also be used in marinades and finishing sauces.

SESAME OIL, made from sesame seeds, also shines with unique healthy qualities. A traditionally used oil in many Asian and Indian cultures, it has grown in popularity in the United States. Dark sesame oil has a stronger flavor and color, complementing soy sauce well, while light is used more as a finishing oil in stir-fries.

- Normalizes blood pressure, reduces cholesterol, and has potent antioxidants
- Helps prevent growth of malignant melanoma, hepatitis, diabetes, and migraines
- Reduces gingivitis-causing bacteria when used as a mouthwash, and destroys strep and other bacteria when gargled
- Alleviates chronic sinusitis when used as nose drops

Sesame oil has a moderate heat tolerance, ideal for sautéing and as finishing sauce. It is enhanced with spices such as basil, garlic, ginger, and peppers.

COCONUT OIL is a highly saturated plant fat, enriching skin and cellular tissue. It's a major player in fending off, or at least keeping at bay, major diseases. Like other plant oils, these medicinal properties apply to pure, unprocessed coconut oil (not hydrogenated coconut oil).

- Improves or even reverses the effects of Alzheimer's, which is now seen as a type 3 form of diabetes. Both type 1 and type 2 diabetes patients benefit from using coconut oil.
- Boosts metabolism and raises body temperatures to promote thyroid health.
- Supports vibrant skin and reduces skin infections and viruses.
- Promotes healthy hair

Since coconut oil is so high in saturated fat, it stays solid at room temperature, but becomes liquid at higher temperatures. Coconut oil has a long shelf life and remains stable in solid or liquid form. To liquefy, place in a bowl of warm water or use another heating method, except the microwave.

The strong tropical scent and flavor serves as a natural sweetener, accenting breads, vegetables, and fruits, and it retains its integrity in high heat for frying, roasting, and baking.

BUTTER AND CHEESE (from grass fed cows)

Imagine grass-fed cows absorbing the rich minerals and vitamin of green grass along with the natural development of sunlight. Now imagine silky, sweet, rich, creamy milk, glowing like the golden sun. That's real butter – and it's bursting with an array of benefits.

Promotes vitamin absorption, and is a great source of Vitamins A, D, E, K, and K2.

- Vitamin D is vital for the immune system; Vitamin E protects our cardiovascular system; Vitamin K helps with blood clotting; and Vitamin A keeps eyes healthy.
- Increases absorption of minerals for a healthy thyroid, adrenals, and other organs. It's a great source of selenium (a super antioxidant) and contains potassium, iodine, and calcium, and keeps calcium from depositing in places it shouldn't (like our cardiovascular system).
- Alleviates gastro-intestinal infection, especially in children and elderly.

- Wards off cancer and strengthens the immune system.
- Butter aids in weight loss and weight management as well as fights against carcinogens.
- Keeps the joints lubricated and mobile.

Look for grass fed or pasture grazed on labels to insure that you're harvesting all of these benefits. A great choice is import butters, such as Kerrygold from Ireland, where cows graze year round.

When you consider how natural oils and fats support wellness, and how processed oils compromise compromise our well-being, it's a no brainer to replace unhealthy fats with those that are good for you, and even taste better. You can find an assortment of pure plant oils at most health food stores, grapeseed and sesame oil at Asian markets, and many grocery stores now stock olive oil, coconut oil, and grass fed butter.

Best Fats for each Blood Type

"O": olive, flaxseed

"A": olive, flaxseed, walnut

"B": olive

"AB": olive, walnut

Health Coach Recommendations

1. Use heat tolerant oils like coconut, grapeseed, and avocado for frying and broiling.
2. Stronger flavored oils can perk up or add a distinct touch to bland foods, such as grains, and enhance vegetables.
3. Add avocados to salads and sandwiches
4. Oils are also medicinal on the skin, scalp, and hair.

Recommended Reading:

Good Fats Cooking, Recipes for a flavor-Packed, Healthy Life by Franklin Becker

Spiritual Reflection of Oil

As water symbolically cleanses us through baptism, so oil symbolically penetrates us for our anointing in the Holy Spirit, by faith, a divine connection. Like an infant that is first washed, then rubbed with oil, leaving its skin soft, smooth, vibrant, flexible, glowing, and shining, so we take in these qualities as the Holy Spirit submerges in us. The Holy Spirit softens our heart with compassion; smooths our crusty edges; revitalizes our spiritual, emotional, and bodily well-being; and makes us glow as shining lights in the midst of darkness.

"You have loved righteousness and hated wickedness; therefore God, your God, has anointed you with the oil of gladness beyond your companions" (Heb. 1:9).

By the *oil of gladness,* we become flexible to respond to the Spirit's intuitive voice. Through this deep penetration, we are *well-oiled*, well able to speak, or that for which we are inspired and led by the Spirit.

Notice how the qualities of physical oil anointing parallel the spiritual anointing.

"So Samuel took the horn of oil and anointed him in the presence of his brothers, and from that day on the Spirit of the Lord came upon David in power" (I Sam. 16:13).

"...God anointed Jesus of Nazareth with the Holy Spirit and power, and how he went around doing good and healing all who were under the power of the devil, because God was with him" (Acts. 10:38).

"They drove out many demons and anointed many sick people with oil and healed them" (Mark 6:13).

"Is anyone among you sick? Let them call the elders of the church to pray over them and anoint them with oil in the name of the Lord" (James 5:14 NIV).

Like the soothing, penetrating qualities of oil, so God's Word pierces even to the bone and marrow, removing pain, depression, and disease.

As we are doused with the oil of the Holy Spirit, we are imbued with the full character of the Spirit. We are free, limitless, and living where God wants us to be, experiencing life in full color. Now born of water and the Spirit, the Christian sees life in the *full color* of God's Truth now revealed by Jesus the Christ.

At Pentecost, the Spirit appeared as tongues of fire. Fire is predominately a combination of the stimulating warming colors of red, yellow, and orange. Thus, we become passionate to do what the Lord has prepared for us. At Christ's baptism, the Spirit appeared as a white dove, symbolizing purity and sanctification. In baptism, we undergo holy baptism upon entrance into the faith life of the Church, and we are set apart from negative baggage and bondage — the Spirit makes us free! The Spirit is also colored as the blue/green water of peace; it is the great comforter and author of life. So we, being renewed at our anointing, show forth the full color of the Holy Spirit.

When the Spirit of the Lord soaks into our hearts, we feel what He feels. He becomes the wind moving our sails in the right place at the right time. He becomes the fire burning so fervently that we cannot help but speak His Words of life. He is the cleansing water bringing peace that surpasses our understanding. We are clothed with His royal robe, and as He is, so are we in this world:

"The spirit of the Lord God is upon me, because the Lord has anointed me; he has sent me to bring good news to the oppressed, to

bind up the brokenhearted, to proclaim liberty to the captives, and release to the prisoners . . . to give them a garland instead of ashes, the oil of gladness instead of mourning, the mantle of praise instead of a faint spirit. They will be called oaks of righteousness, the planting of the LORD, to display his glory" (Isaiah 61:1,3 ISV).

Finally, we come to the last category of the pyramid, protein, which like oils, is crucial yet controversial. The science of blood type explains why some thrive more on animal protein, while others do well with more vegetable protein.

Perfect Protein

What makes a protein perfect is that it's perfect for you. Since no one diet fits all, it's beneficial to be familiar with a variety of proteins to intuitively choose what you need at any given time.

As we become sensitive to our natural nutritional instinct, we may have cravings for certain proteins. For instance, you might crave a less healthy food which contains dairy, like ice cream or a processed meat. Sometimes, we are craving the protein, not necessarily all the sugar or flavorings. Therefore, understanding the protein need behind the cravings can help us be satisfied with healthier choices, although it's wise to leave a little margin to eat ice cream or whatever you desire. This is called the 90/10 rule: eat healthily 90% of the time to allow anything else in the remaining 10% (unless a strict diet is medically required). This rule helps us maintain balance and a good relationship with food. Here are three considerations for the amount and protein type.

How much protein helps you thrive? Too much protein can cause organ and bone damage, while too little prevents overall development and growth. Notice that the Science of Nutrition Pyramid recommends about 25 - 30% protein, a smaller portion than the government pyramid allows. Equally important is the quality of protein, which creates an environment for robust health or sickness.

What forms of protein is best for you? Some thrive on a vegan or vegetarian diet, others don't. Everyone has different protein needs.

Type "A" blood types tend to do well on more vegetarian protein, due to their agrarian evolution. The key to well-balanced nutrition on a vegan or vegetarian diet is variety. Properly planned, it is nutritionally satisfying and promotes numerous health benefits including a reduced risk of heart disease, colon and lung cancer, osteoporosis, diabetes, kidney disease, hypertension, obesity, and a number of other debilitating conditions. Poorly planned, however, it can result in low vitamin deficiency especially B12, and lead to sugar cravings. The following plant based proteins will help add diversity to your protein pallet so that your mammal instinct readily selects just what it needs.

The Nutty Profile

Nuts and seeds are concentrated sources, full of protein, good fats, vitamins, iron, magnesium, and other minerals, with many health benefits.

Clue 1. *Notice how a walnut looks like the upper and lower cerebrum?* Indeed, walnuts nourish the brain and adrenal glands, are high in protein and iron, and contain omega 3 fatty acids. They reduce inflammation and pain, and lubricate the lungs and intestines.

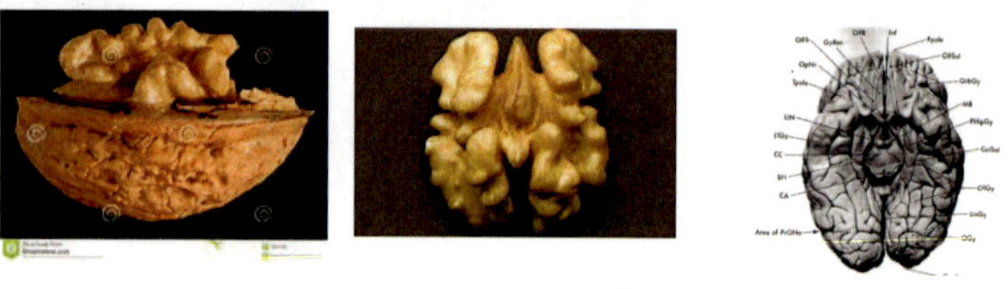

Clue 2. *See how the grain lines in almonds continuously wrap around it?* Almonds provide continuous grains of energy and fortify us with high minerals including calcium, magnesium, potassium, and iron.

Clue 3. *Sunflower seeds are one of the rare plant sources of the sunshine vitamin D.* They are also high in protein, unsaturated fats, phosphorus, calcium, iron, fluorine, iodine, potassium, magnesium, zinc, B vitamins, and vitamin E.

- Pumpkin seeds help eliminate intestinal parasites such as roundworm and tapeworm. They are also used to treat impotence and prostate enlargement due to their high zinc content.
- Cashews are energizing, help maintain healthy gums and teeth, support good cardiovascular health, eliminate free radicals, and support healthy muscles and bones. They also helps promote normal sleep patterns in menopausal women.
- Pecans are bountiful in antioxidants and protein with over 19 vitamins and minerals.
- Sesame seeds are high in calcium, magnesium, niacin, vitamins A and E, and protein.
- Brazil nuts are an abundant source of selenium, an antioxidant that boosts immunity.
- Flaxseeds are the richest source of omega 3 fatty acids, improving immunity and reducing high cholesterol. Flaxseed meal effectively prevents constipation and has antitumor and antioxidant properties. Flaxseeds also help balance estrogen levels. However, there are some who are gluten-intolerant (not all) who find that flax seed causes constipation so must avoid this seed.
- Hazelnuts are rich in calcium, magnesium, iron, potassium, phosphorus, folic acid, vitamin E, and strengthen the stomach.
- Pistachio nuts purify the blood, lubricate the intestines, and treat constipation.
- Peanuts are a legume and, like nuts, are rich in many vitamins, iron, zinc, and protein.

Nuts and seeds are the perfect *convenience food* chock full of nutrition. Blend your favorite nuts in little baggies for a quick boost of protein.

For those having difficulty digesting nuts and seeds, for variety try nut and seed bi-products, such as nut milk and nut butter which contain the same nutritional value as nuts, so long as they're not overly processed.

Health Benefits of Nut Milk

Nut milk is an excellent healthy alternative to cow's milk, with many nutritional benefits.

Nut milk is lactose-free. Those who are lactose intolerant (can't metabolize the lactose sugar found in cow's milk), do well with nut milk. It is also gluten-free so individuals with gluten allergies or celiac disease can also enjoy it and experience this healthy, rich, creamy natural beverage. Below are three common nut milks containing about 50% more calcium than cow's milk! The Coconut/Almond, blend now at most grocers is a delicious balance of rich, creamy, and sweet with the combined nutrition of both milks. Alternately, homemade nut milk kits can be ordered on sites such as wheatgrasskits.com.

- Almond milk is rich in protein, calcium, potassium, and magnesium.
- Coconut milk is full of protein, calcium, and vitamin D.
- Cashew milk is abundant in protein, potassium, magnesium, and vitamin A.

Butter up with Nut Butter

Wholesome nut spreads contain a host of minerals, vitamins, and fiber, offering good-quality, usable protein that are a good tasty replacement for margarine or processed spreads.

Nut butters are good for children (without nut allergies). Replacing commercial nut spreads (containing hydrogenated fats) with nutritious all natural nut butters provides essential protein for health and growth. Spread nut butters on toast, bagels, waffles, and pancakes. *The Nut Butter Cookbook* by Robin Robertson demonstrates 100 delicious vegan recipes made with nut butter.

What a great protein for distinct, rich flavor enhancement! Some common nut and seed butters include the following:

- almond butter
- cashew butter
- hazelnut butter
- sesame seed butter
- sunflower seed butter
- peanut butter

These butters can be found in most health food stores. Both nut milks and nut butters allow you to reap the same nutritional value as the nut itself in many enjoyable ways.

Best Nuts and Seeds for each Blood Type

"**O**": walnut, pumpkin seed, flaxseed

"**A**": walnut, pumpkin seed, peanut, flaxseed

"**B**": walnut

"**AB**": chestnut, walnut, peanut

- Chew nuts well for easy digestion. This is very important because most of our energy is used for digestion.
- Choose raw nuts because roasting depletes nutrition.
- Consume limited amounts if weight loss is desired. They are rich in omega 3 fatty acids, however, which can actually improve metabolism.
- Try nut bi-products for variety and easy digestion.

Bountiful Beans and Legumes

Beans are a bounty of plant-based protein, high in iron, B vitamins, fiber, and are quite versatile. Like nuts, the nutritious by-products, such as humus, bean dip, and tofu, offer variety and easy digestibility, as do desserts like black bean brownies. Beans can also be placed in small containers and frozen. You can create a bean bank, like the grain bank, and make deposits with excess leftover beans.

A few challenges with beans are that they can be time consuming to cook and difficult to digest. Here are some tips.

- Use a pressure cooker to reduce cooking time.
- Soak beans, changing the water as needed.
- Chew beans thoroughly to help assimilate the nutritional value.
- Smaller beans are easier to digest, like adzuki, lentils, mung beans, and peas.
- Legumes are best with green or non-starchy vegetables.
- Season with unrefined sea salt or soy sauce toward the end of cooking. If salt is added at the beginning, the beans won't fully cook. Salt also helps digestion.
- Adding fennel or cumin near the end of cooking helps prevent gas.
- Pour a little apple cider, brown rice, or white wine vinegar into the water in the last stages of cooking to soften the beans, making them more digestible.

Once again, cookbooks can inspire new flavors and pizzazz to this otherwise bland, but extremely nutritious, food. Here are two: *Bean by Bean* by Crescent Dragonwagon, and *The Better Bean Cookbook* by Jenny Chandler.

Best Beans and Legumes for each Blood Type

"O": black-eyed peas, adzuki beans

"A": black bean, adzuki bean, black-eyed peas, green beans, lentil, pinto bean, soybean

"B": kidney bean, lima bean, navy bean

"AB": lentil, navy bean, pinto bean, soy bean

You might not think of grains, greens, and fruit as protein foods, but here are many containing moderate to high amounts of protein:

Greens: peas, kale, broccoli, mushroom, corn, artichokes, spinach, collard greens, parsley, mustard greens, zucchini, beet greens, arugula, brussel sprouts, and bamboo shoots.

Grains: wheat germ, wheat bran, oats, oat bran, brown rice, rice bran, spelt, kamut, quinoa, and amaranth.

Fruits: avocados, bananas, cherries, kiwi fruit, guavas, apricots, blackberries, raspberries, strawberries, nectarines, passion fruit, pomegranates, and oranges.

There is certainly a wide spectrum of plant-based protein, and the key to a healthy plant-based diet is to draw from these varieties to help you feel nutritionally satisfied. These amazing cookbooks can help make even bland proteins, like tofu, deliciously satisfying as well.

Animal Protein

The quality, quantity, and type of animal protein are determining factors in creating health. Naturally grazed and raised animals have a much higher nutritional value and without the antibiotics and emotional trauma of living in unnatural conditions. We absorb all of these elements when we consume animal meat. Here is where you are what you eat actually becomes literal!

First, what type is right for your blood type? Blood type "O" has the strongest stomach acid, designed to break down animal protein and assimilate well. This stems from their hunter/gatherer evolution when this was the main game. Type "B" also digests animal protein well, but favors certain animals, as outlined in all types at the end of this section. Type "A" is limited due to a more delicate digestive system.

Second, small amounts, such as five to seven ounces per meal, adequately meets nutritional requirements without taxing the bodily systems.

Third, quality animal protein optimizes our well-being, while unnaturally grazed animals yield disease. While naturally bred animals cost more, a smaller portion is adequate due to their higher nutritional profile, as seen below.

Grass Fed VS. Grain Fed

Animals that are grass fed take in the nourishment of direct sunshine and the rich minerals of grass, as we do, when we eat dark green leafy vegetables. Pasture grazed animals also absorb their environment of freedom, fresh air, and harmony with nature, without antibiotics and pesticides. We, too, are imbued with those qualities when consuming them. Grass Fed, also called Pasture Fed, meat is a great value, considering so many benefits, even though it costs more.

Best Meat for each Blood Type

"O": beef, lamb, liver, veal, venison, buffalo, mutton

"A": chicken, Cornish hens, turkey

"B": goat, lamb, mutton, rabbit, venison

"AB": goat, lamb, mutton, rabbit, liver, pheasant

Wild Salmon VS. Farmed Salmon (and other fish)

Salmon is known for its health benefits. It's delicious and easy to prepare in a variety of ways. Since wild salmon has been over-fished, salmon farms have been sprouting up to make the fish more widely available and affordable. In salmon farms, operators control the production and feed while fish are confined to a certain area by nets. Farmed salmon have significantly higher levels of pesticides, mercury, and other carcinogens than wild salmon, but are less expensive and available year round. Wild salmon retains greater nutrition and is much less contaminated, yet is pricey and seasonal. Recently, wild caught has become more affordable. Again, a smaller quantity of a higher quality is a better value in all ways.

Best Seafood for each Blood Type

"O": bass, cod, halibut, red snapper, perch, shad, sole, swordfish, yellowtail

"A": cod, mackerel, perch, pollack, red snapper, salmon, sardine, trout, whiting

"B": caviar, cod, croaker, flounder, haddock, halibut, perch, salmon, sardine, sole

"AB": cod, croaker, mackerel, mahi-mahi, red snapper, salmon, sardine, shad, tuna

Dairy Products

Butter, cheese, and milk that comes from naturally grazed animals with the least amount of processing will retain the rich, pasture-fed mineral source. The full-bodied color, taste, and texture of organic fed animals are not only deliciously creamy, but they promote better nutritional absorption. It also eliminates growth hormones that are frequently used in the *meat market,* which are passed along to human consumption. Pasture fed dairy contains five times greater conjugated linoleic acid (CLA), shown to protect the heart and aid in weight loss, and is higher in vitamin D3 and omega-3 fatty acids.

Blood Type "B" and "AB" are well suited for a variety of dairy products, since dairy foods were first introduced in the Type "B" era with the domestication of animals. All other types should be limited to a modest consumption.

Best Dairy for each Blood Type

"O": butter; eggs; mozzarella, feta, farmer, and goat cheese; ghee

"A": eggs; mozzarella, feta, farmer, ricotta, and goat cheese; goat milk; ghee; yogurt

"B": cow/goat milk; cottage, ricotta, farmer, feta, and goat cheese; kefir; yogurt

"AB": goat milk; cottage, mozzarella, ricotta, farmer, feta, and goat cheese; sour cream; yogurt

In conclusion of this various array of protein, your perfect proteins are a variety that agree with your blood type. Sometimes, we get stuck on a certain food, but it's important to tune in to our inner mammal to direct us to our protein needs.

The following observation is an interesting and humorous phenomenon of the saying, "*You are what you eat.*" Literally!

Energetics of Animal Food

As we reap specific energetic qualities of plant foods when we eat them, so we can take on the energetic qualities of animals when we consume the same animal meat *continually for years*, a theory called *cross-species transference* (merging with the energetic character of an animal). Here are a few examples of these energetic traits in specific animals.

In almost every culture, there is some form of chicken soup for the sick. Why chicken? It's not the nutritional properties of chicken, but rather its energetic qualities. What is the essential character of a chicken? A chicken is lively, spunky, and vital. As we consume chicken, we are imbued with these very qualities, which is what we need to recover.

What is the essential character of a cow? A cow is a big, sturdy, heavy animal. Why do men tend to eat more beef? This is complementary to a man's bulkier, heavier build, providing strength and stability. The red meat has high protein and is insulating with heating properties, having a warm moist effect due to fat and blood.

What is the essential character of a deer? It is agile, has sharp senses, and is very fast. This was a primary animal that Indians ate, and these were the very characteristics that they needed for their own survival. In this sense, they became what they ate.

In addition to the essential character of the animal is the animal's natural temperature and moisture. Compare a duck to a chicken. A duck is very oily, making it quite moist, and the oil insulates it well, making it durable even in cold weather. Therefore, it has a natural moist, warming effect on us as we consume it. A chicken, on the other hand, is much drier, and has a cooling effect.

Therefore, if we are naturally a hot blooded, hot tempered type, we might consider eating meat with a cooling effect to help us maintain balance or warm insulating properties if we are naturally cold. Below are a few pictures just for fun and to demonstrate this phenomenon that we truly *are what we eat (continuously)*. Observe their face and whole body, and guess what animal they raise or hunt.

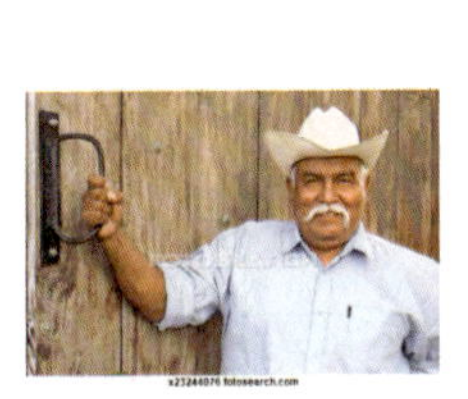

Cattleman

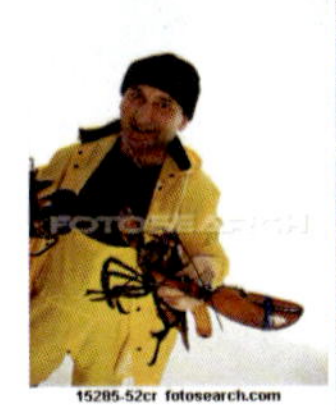

Fisherman

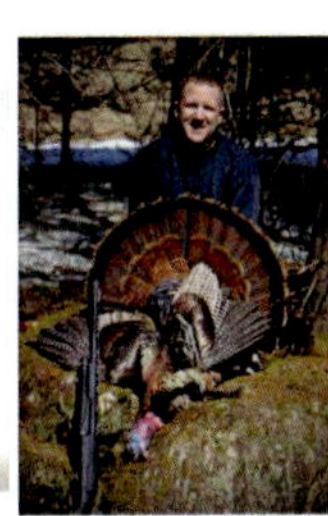

Turkey hunter

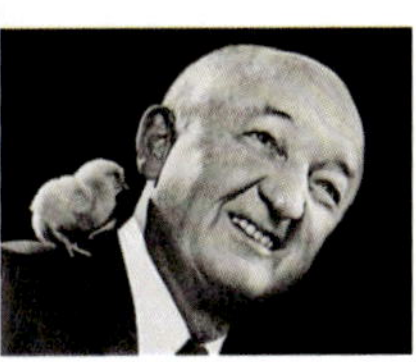

Frank Perdue

<u>Health Coach Recommendations:</u>

- Enjoy a variety of protein sources for a broad spectrum of health benefits.
- Eat high quality, but small quantity, of proteins at a time.

- Use cookbooks to learn how to make sauces, soups, and stews that can make bland foods pop.
- Consume the proteins that are right for you and understand that cravings are sometimes intuitively directing towards certain proteins.

Recommended Reading:

The Great Vegan Protein Book by Celine Steen and Tamasin Noyes
The Nut Butter Cookbook by Robin Robertson

Beans and nuts in the following Spiritual Reflection spotlight two primary foods in biblical times as seen in these spiritual reflections.

Spiritual Reflection of Beans in the Bible

Take thou also unto thee wheat and barley and beans and lentils, and millet, and fitches, and put them into one vessel, and make thee bread thereof... (Ezekiel 4:9 KJV).

This recipe is referred to as "Ezekiel's bread," which the seizure prophet gave to prepare for the seize of Jerusalem. It's no wonder, with all of their healing qualities, that beans are primary ingredients.

As reported in 2nd Samuel, beans were among the highly nutritious foods sent to feed King David's hungry army and restore strength… wheat and barley and meal, and parched corn, and beans, and lentils, and parched pulse... *They also brought wheat and barley, flour and roasted grain, beans and lentils, honey and curds, sheep, and cheese from cows' milk for David and his people to eat. For they said, 'The people have become exhausted and hungry and thirsty in the wilderness* (2 Samuel 17:28-29 NIV).

Beans were a wonderful source of protein - a scarce commodity in primitive times, full of vitamin C, iron, and dietary fiber which helps lower LDL, reduces blood pressure, and helps control insulin and blood sugar levels, vital to the health of diabetics.

They also inhibit the growth of cancer, containing a substance that converts into a kind of natural chemotherapy chemical that searches through the body for cancer indicators to deactivate it.

Beans are nature's regulators. They are a quick and effective cure for constipation by keeping wastes moving along at a regular, healthy pace, reducing the risks of colon or rectal cancer, intestinal disorders, and hemorrhoids.

Ezekiel bread is still alive and well today, *literally!* Due to its sprouting process, it is a live food with many beneficial enzymes. Sprouted seed breads are easily digestible for blood Type "O."

And alongside the torrent there will come up, along its bank on this side and on that side, all sorts of trees for food..... And their fruitage must prove to be for food and their leafage for healing (Ezekiel 47:12 NWT).

<u>Spiritual Reflection of Almonds in the Bible</u>

The word of the LORD came to me: "What do you see, Jeremiah?" "I see the branch of an almond tree," I replied. The LORD said to me, "You have seen correctly, for I am watching to see that my word is fulfilled" (Jeremiah 1:12).

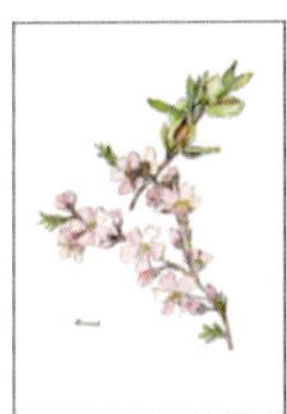
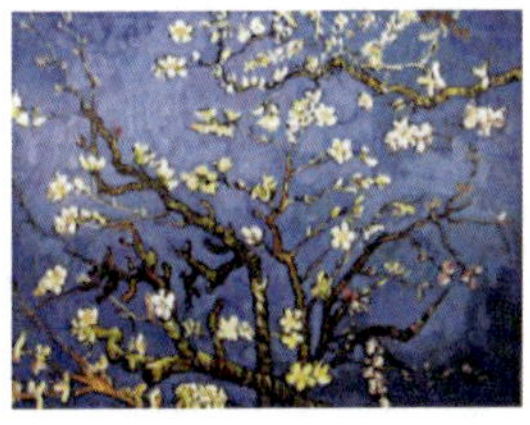
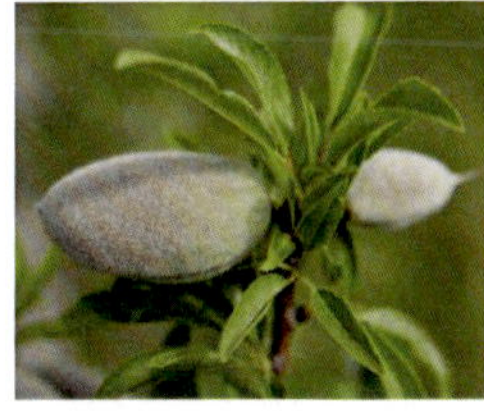

The almond tree blooms earlier than any other flowering tree, as early as February, with beautiful light pink blossoms which appear before the leaves. The early blossoming is why the Hebrew word for *almond* means "awakening and watching."

God calls upon Jeremiah to be a witness for God, but initially he protests the position God is calling him into...for Jeremiah says, "Ah, Lord God! Behold, I do not know how to speak, for I am a youth" (Jer. 1:6 NASB). In fact, Jeremiah was but a *budding youth,* only 18 years old, considered too young for service within the Levitical priesthood. Nevertheless, the Lord tells Jeremiah that he will speak the Word of the Lord clearly and authoritatively to the people of Israel and even to Israel's enemies who will be drafted by God in a grand plan to awaken Israel that she may return to the Lord.

Likewise, Aaron, Moses' brother, was called to be the spokesman before Pharaoh and became the High Priest for the Israelites during the Exodus from Egypt. As a sign that God would be with them, Aaron's staff of Almond wood bloomed..

"The next day Moses entered the Tent of the Testimony and saw that Aaron's staff, which represented the house of Levi, had not only sprouted but had budded, blossomed, and produced almonds" (Numbers 17:8 HCSB).

Aaron's staff was later placed in the Ark of the Covenant, a sign of the miraculous work of God. So, the *almond wood*, and therefore almonds, from a biblical point of view, hold symbolic meaning of God's presence with the Prophet/Priest, the people of Israel, and ultimately, for all people. Thus, when God asks Jeremiah to say what he sees, Jeremiah's response about seeing the almond tree becomes a Hebrew play on words...for the word almond means *watch, see, and awaken.*

Jeremiah is anointed by God to be a great Prophet in the Line of Aaron the priest — and the living Word of God will become visible to him through the imagery of the almond branch. In our vernacular, God asked, "Jeremiah, what do you see?"

"A walking stick," I said. "Yes, you see well that I am *walking* with you and will make every word *stick!*"

Almonds also appear in the story of Joseph as part of the gift from his father.

"Then their father Israel said to them, 'If it must be, then do this: Put some of the best products of the land in your bags and take them down to the man as a gift—a little balm and a little honey, some spices and myrrh, some pistachio nuts and almonds'" (Genesis 43:11).

Almonds are still prized for their crunchy texture and smooth taste, enhancing and complementing many foods. They are also admired for their aesthetic beauty as the shape of jewelry in necklace and earring pendants and dangling chandelier crystals. This was the shape the Lord commanded for His furnishings.

"Three cups shaped like almond flowers with buds and blossoms were on one branch, three on the next branch, and the same for all six branches extending from the lampstand. And on the lampstand were four cups shaped like almond flowers with buds and blossoms" (Exodus 37: 19, 20).

The delicate almond branch, with early lovely inflorescence, leaves a powerful impression of God's presence awakening in our lives. The Lord is preparing us for blossoming even when the bud is not yet visible during our winter season. In the dormant season, we are often awakened by challenges that eventually become fruitful opportunities. The Lord is walking with us. He is watching over His word. It will be fulfilled as it sticks with us.

Look closely at almonds and see how each has unique grain lines, like artfully curved brush strokes, across the whole nut. Perhaps this is how God sees us, as His Almond Joy!

Herbs and Spices

Finally, a complementary category of the pyramid is *herbs and spices.* While this is not actually one of the groups, it enhances all of the food groups and is medicinal for each blood type. Therefore, we complete the pyramid with a dash or a douse of condiments. Spices and seasonings can actually improve digestion and immunity. The following are the specific ones to support and enhance each blood type.

Type O need plenty of Iodine to help regulate the thyroid gland and the metabolic process for weight control. Kelp is a rich source and kelp-based seasonings (found in most health food stores) are a flavorful way to add it to dishes. Natural Salt is another good source, but use it sparingly.

Parsley helps soothe the digestive tract. Warming spices such as curry and cayenne pepper also help digestion. Turmeric, known as a great anti-inflammatory, is also ideal for Type "O" with inflammation vulnerabilities, such as arthritis.

Type A especially need immune boosters. Soy-based spices are especially good, such as soy sauce and tamari.

Blackstrap molasses, a rich source of iron, compensates for the primary vegetarian protein of the Type A diet. Garlic and parsley is also recommended, and kelp for its iodine and minerals.

Type B does well with parsley and warming herbs like ginger, curry, and cayenne pepper.

Type AB also needs iodine in the form of sea salt and kelp. Soy sauce and garlic are also good.

Best Herbs/Spices for each Blood Type

"O": kelp, parsley, curry, cayenne pepper, and turmeric

"A": soy sauce, tamari, blackstrap molasses, and kelp

"B": parsley, ginger, curry, and cayenne pepper

"AB": sea salt, kelp, soy sauce, and garlic

Spiritual Reflection of Herbs and Spices

Herbs and spices in biblical times were presented as luxury gifts to honor royalty or those highly esteemed, such as Solomon's lover. They were used to worship, honor, and anoint Jesus; these special herbs, spices, and oils escorted our Lord through his birth, death, and resurrection.

"After coming into the house, they saw the Child with Mary His mother; and they fell to the ground and worshiped Him. Then, opening their treasures, they presented to Him gifts of gold, frankincense, and myrrh" (Matthew 2:11 NASB).

Frankincense is a fragrant aroma that was used during ceremonial offerings and considered an article of luxury. What a fitting spice for the greatest ceremony to the earth – the birth of our Savior!

Frankincense medicinal uses include antidepressant, anti-stress, and a powerful inflammation remedy now known as Boswellia. It is also a primary ingredient in arthritis relief. They presented this gift as they bowed down to worship Him!

In Biblical times, Myrrh is the anointing oil used in the Tabernacle for purification. It was considered a natural remedy for almost every human affliction. What an amazing reflection of what Jesus came to be for humankind!

"Then Mary took about a pint of pure nard, an expensive perfume; she poured it on Jesus' feet and wiped his feet with her hair. And the house was filled with the fragrance of the perfume" (John 12:3).

Mary, Lazarus' sister, pours a pint of pure nard to anoint Jesus' feet (worth about a year's wages). When Judas protests (ironically, the one who eventually sells Jesus), Jesus subtly responds that there is no monetary value that can be placed on the time he will be presented and revealed as Lord and Savior. Mary also *poured* her whole self unto the Lord; not only offering the extravagant oil, but her tears and hair as a sign of adoration and appreciation for the Savior. The offering of ourselves as we surrender in personal devotion to God is a sweet smelling savor unto the Lord. Our love is as perfume and extravagant spices — bringing out the flavors Christ elicits from us. You, in the completeness of who you are, are of much worth!

Nard was an intensely aromatic, amber-colored, thick oil used as a perfume. Nard is a natural sedative that relieves insomnia, anxiety, and even birthing difficulties. Mary anointed Jesus' feet; feet symbolically carry the Gospel of liberty, releasing all from fear. She demonstrated her priceless love for our Savior just days before the Passover, which would begin the chain of events leading to his costly sacrifice for our new birth.

At the crucifixion, a hyssop branch was offered for medicinal purposes.

"Nicodemus, who had first come to Him by night, also came, bringing a mixture of myrrh and aloes, about a hundred pounds weight" (John 19:29 NASB).

Symbolically hyssop was used as a cleansing herb. This was offered to Jesus, and his blood *cleansed* us.

"Purge me with hyssop, and I shall be clean; wash me, and I shall be whiter than snow" (Psalm 51:7 KJV).

"A jar of sour wine was sitting there, so they soaked a sponge in it, put it on a hyssop branch, and held it up to his lips" (John 19:29 ESV).

Finally, burial spices were brought to anoint Jesus body.

The cleansing spice, Myrrh, *considered a natural remedy for almost every human affliction,* was used in both the birth and burial of our Lord. It was used with the embalming aloes in preserving the Lord's body, which fulfilled another prophesy:

"For Thou wilt not leave my soul in hell; neither wilt Thou suffer Thine Holy One to see corruption" (Psalm 16:10 KJV).

By the addition of the herbs and spices that anointed Him, our Lord fulfilled our complete redemption. May we forever worship and honor him with our whole being and extravagant love for Him. He has fully cleansed us and relieves our *every human affliction.*

If you look back to the Science of Nutrition Pyramid, notice under the pyramid is the most vital element that supports our whole well-being – water.

Water – the Spring of Wellness

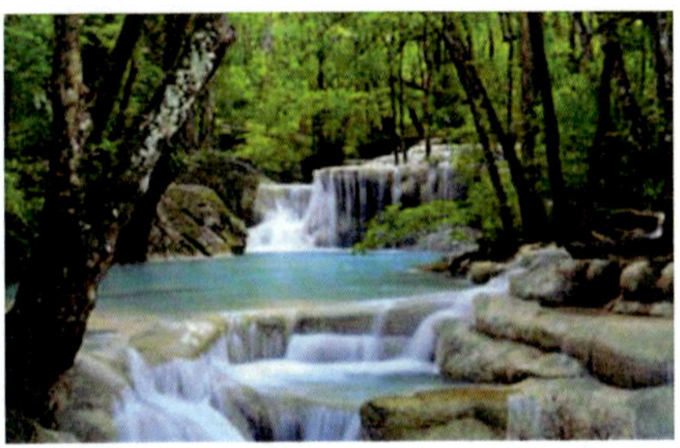

While water has no nutritional value, it is essential to produce energy and helps assimilate nutrition. You can survive without eating for weeks, but only a few days without water. Ideally, we should drink half of our body weight in ounces. For instance, a 130 lb. person should drink 65 oz. of water daily (about a half-gallon). There are three primary reasons why water is so crucial.

First, mild dehydration declines our mental speed and can lead to headaches and even arthritis. Dr. F. Batmaghelidj, an expert on water, points out that the body has no water storage system to draw on in time of need. The areas of our body most acutely affected by a water shortage are areas without a direct blood supply, such as cartilage in the joints. Painful joints, including arthritis, can be the result of inadequate water intake. Severe dehydration contributes to a host of serious and chronic disease.

Dr. F. Batmaghelidj explains why water works so well in keeping us healthy and pain free and can even cure illnesses. Water is the basis of all life. Your muscles that move your body are *75% water;* your blood that transports nutrients is *82% water*; your lungs that provide your oxygen are *90% water;* your brain that is the control center of your body is *76% water*; and even your bones are *25% water.*

Second, water is essential to flush out toxins. Some toxins are environmental, such as the air we breathe and the food we eat, but the majority are formed inside the body as normal waste products, which accumulate rapidly. Without adequate water, our bodies can't flush out the toxins fast enough, resulting in decreased energy, impaired organ function, and ultimately, disease.

Thirst is not necessarily an indicator of dehydration. The body retains fluids in a state of dehydration to compensate for the lack of water. When this happens, we retain toxic fluids that we're supposed to eliminate. This increases the level of toxins in your tissues, inviting chronic disease and premature aging. Water also hydrates our skin with a healthy glow and flexibility.

Third, water is vital in maintaining proper body temperature. Your body's ability to cool itself depends on adequate water intake. High fevers are often associated with dehydration, and doctors usually recommend drinking plenty of water for fever. Water is like coolant in your car. Low levels can cause overheating.

Finally, the quality of water is just as important as quantity. Tap water is often contaminated by chlorine, hard minerals, heavy metals, and pesticides. This seems somewhat counterproductive, since water is supposed to help us detoxify.

Tap water should be purified or distilled, as should bottled water, even if labeled as spring water, drinking water, or mineral water. Like plants, we need much water to be colorful, energetic, and vibrant.

Health Coach Recommendations:

- Drink a full glass of water in the morning prior to any food or drink. This helps to flush out the toxins from the overnight internal cleansing.
- Install a quality water filter under your sink for cooking, etc.
- Many beverages such as coffee, soda, energy drinks, and alcohol are dehydrating. Gradually replace with more water – the real energy drink!
- Too much water can cause mineral imbalance and disrupt sleep.

- Too little water can cause headaches, fatigue, hunger, sugar cravings, etc.
- Add citrus (lemon/lime) to drinking water for daily cleansing and flavor.
- Try drinking only water with your meals for a week - feel the many benefits.

Recommended Reading:

Your Body's Many Cries for Water by Dr. F. Batmaghelidj

Spiritual Reflection of Water in the Bible

And the Spirit of God moved upon the face of the waters (Gen. 1:2 AKJV).

The Spirit of God flows upon many waters through the holy scriptures, rippling in rich imagery and meaning. Let's sail on this spiritually symbolic journey together!

In Genesis, the garden of Eden was watered by rivers, enriching plants, animals, and humans.

And God said, Let the waters bring forth abundantly the moving creatures that hath life, and fowl that may fly above the earth in the open firmament of heaven (Gen. 1:20 KJV).

All life emanates from water. As the water *brings forth life* in the beginning, so a baby is born when the mother's water *breaks forth with life.* Jesus further compares the physical birth with spiritual birth, in John 3:5 KJV:

"Except a man be born of water and of the Spirit, he cannot enter into the kingdom of God."

Jesus takes Nicodemus (and all who have ears to hear) deeper into the living water, where it cleanses, purifies, and sanctifies us.

"That he might sanctify and cleanse it (the church) with the washing of water by the word" (Eph. 5:26 KJV).

"Wherewithal shall a young man cleanse his way… by taking heed thereto according to thy word" (Psalm 119:9 AKJV).

God's word cleanses us by meditating on it and speaking it. From John 13:9 (KJV), we learn that Jesus further demonstrated this purification by washing his disciple's feet.

"Simon Peter saith unto him, Lord, (wash) not my feet only, but also my hands and my head. Jesus saith to him, He that is washed needeth not save to wash his feet, but is clean every whit: and ye are clean, but not all."

Here Jesus brings in another dimension, foreshadowing the complete purification through baptism of the Holy Spirit. Peter really gets it, a *deep cleaning,* and perhaps in a joking, yet dead serious look in his eyes, he was saying, *"Lord, not just my feet, but shower me with all that you are."* He also instructs them to wash each other's feet. Feet symbolically carry the gospel.

"How beautiful on the mountains are the feet of those who bring good news…" (Isaiah 52:7).

"Whoever does not receive you, nor heed your words, as you go out of that house or that city, shake the dust off your feet" (Matt: 10:14 NASB).

Thus, we wash each other's feet by sharing the cleansing word of God. Furthermore, we are to shake off the dust of doubt when we depart an unbelieving environment.

Moses was instructed to make a washing basin in the tabernacle where the priests could wash their hands and feet that they die not, that they could be purified. *"Thou shalt also make a laver of brass, and his foot also of brass, to wash withal: and thou shalt put it between the tabernacle of the congregation and the altar, and thou shalt put water therein"* (Ex: 30:18 KJV).

Similarly, we are washed from the world's debris of negative thoughts and emotions. *"Now ye are clean through the word which I have spoken to you"* (John 15:3 KJV).

Beyond cleansing, water is also a reflecting pool of perfect peace. *"He makes me lie down in green pastures. He leads me beside still waters"* (Psalms 23:2 NLV).

On the flip side, He stills the raging waters. *"And he awoke and rebuked the wind and said to the sea, 'Peace! Be still!' And the wind ceased, and there was a great calm"* (Mark 4:39 ESV).

Sometimes He calms the turbulent waters of life and other times He calls us to walk over it - with Him: *"Yes, come," Jesus said. So Peter went over the side of the boat and walked on the water toward Jesus* (Matthew 14:29 NLT).

The Lord rows us to a place of security and serenity, whether He guides us to still waters, calms our raging waters, or causes us to walk on top of the stormy seas. Ultimately, He takes us to our eternal home where there is no more turbulent seas. *"And I saw a new heaven and a new earth: for the first heaven and the first earth were passed away; and there was no more sea"* (Rev.21:1 KJV).

Finally, water is also a transformative provision, such as when Jesus turns the water used for ceremonial washing into the grandest of all wine. Similarly, Jesus, as the *Living Water that has come down from heaven*, changes our insufficiencies into rich, grand wonders. When we drink of the everlasting water, we will not thirst, we will not want. As our Lord said to the woman he met by the well: *"But whosoever drinketh of the water that I shall give him shall never thirst; but the water that I shall give him shall be in him a well of water springing up into everlasting life"* (John 4:14 KJV).

Water is the birthing and rebirthing of all of creation. It is the well spring of life, refreshing, cleansing, and purifying. Upon our turbulent seas, He bids us to come and walk on water. He is the eternal water that flows forever.

This concludes the science of nutrition coinciding with the science of blood type. We now open another genesis gem, *seasons,* reflected in body types and the daily cycle.

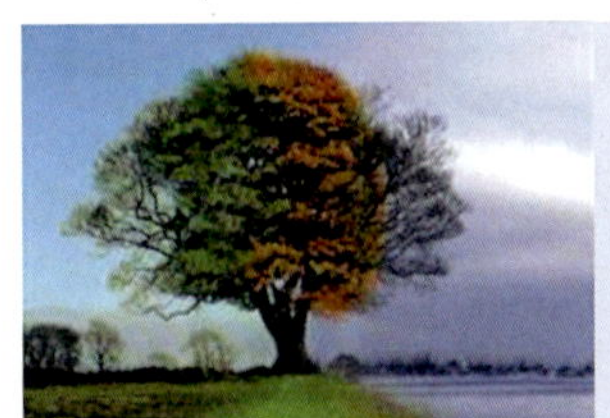

CHAPTER 8

Best Lifestyle for Your Body and Emotional Type

Then God said, *"Let lights appear in the sky to separate the day from the night. Let them be signs to mark the seasons, days, and years"* (Gen: 1:14 NLT).

What an amazing perspective of our loving Creator's multi-dimensional structures! Lights - not only separating day from night, but in the grand plan, bring meaning to our lives, continuity to our time, and once again, health to our well-being. Here we'll see not only time marked by transitions, but how *we too* are marked by seasons, physically and emotionally.

The holistic medicinal arts used traditionally in India, correlate the science of life with three seasons: winter (Vata), spring (Kapha), and summer (Pita). These three seasons are also reflected in daily cycles, and body types. As we synchronize with these seasons, we naturally achieve greater balance and health.

In the daily cycle, *Kapha* marks the *spring* time of day from 6 a.m. to 10 a.m. Like the spring season with heavy rains that wash away winter debris, our bodies begin elimination from our night time cleansing, which is why drinking water is essential in the morning. In the morning, our bodies are stronger and heavier, making it the best time for physical activity.

Then, *we* move to *Pitta,* the *summer* time of day, from 10 a.m. to 2 p.m. This is when digestion is strongest. By consuming most food during this period, while digestion is cranking, we best metabolize and utilize what we consume. It's the optimal time for heavier foods and protein. Ideally, consume about 60% of daily food during this period.

Finally, *Vata,* the *winter* time of day from 2 p.m. to 6 p.m. is when the mind is most alert and mental production should be at its peak. Mental vitality during this time is primed by adhering to the needs of the previous periods, such as exercise in the morning and adequate food consumption in midday.

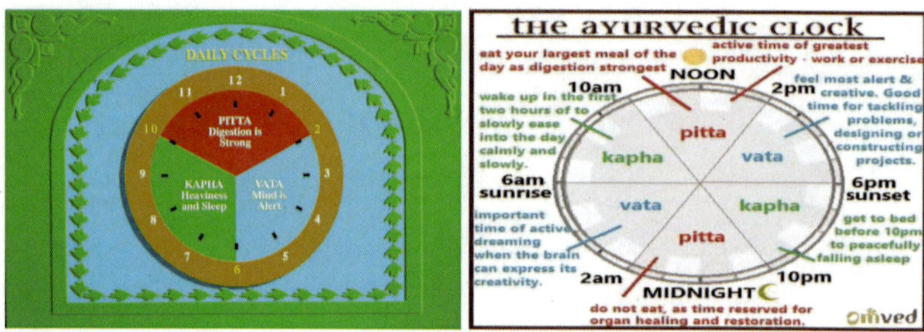

Conversely, as we move into the second phase of the Ayurvedic clock, we begin the polar transitions.

Kapha, from 6 p.m. to 10 p.m., is when we gradually decrease physical activity and food (after evening meal). The target time for bed to harmonize with this natural cycle is 10 p.m.

Pitta resumes from 10 p.m. to 2 a.m., the time to *refrain* from eating, when digestion and all organs need to rest and recover from daily stress.

Vata recommences from 2 a.m. to 6 a.m. when the brain is in active dream mode. Creativity is cresting with the sunrise, especially as we are aligned with nature's patterns.

When we harmonize with these daily patterns, we soar with the nature's *jet wind*, with vitality, creativity, and weight management, among many benefits. While we are all greatly affected by these natural daily *tides,* each individual also reflects a certain season according to their individual body and emotional type.

As we define our appearance in terms of seasons, such as summer blondes, fall auburns, and winter brunettes, with correlating skin tones, our *season* helps us determine the best colors and shades to complement our own unique beauty. Similarly, the season of our body type and emotional type, helps us determine the best food and lifestyle to enhance our wellness.

Consider your body type and emotional type. For instance, I have a Kapha emotional type and a Pitta body. You may well recognize your type from the description below. Each body type correlates with certain earth elements, characteristics, strengths, and weaknesses.

A *Kapha* body type is a big bone, large body frame. The Kapha dosha (body or mind type) elements are *earth and water.* The nature of Kapha tends to reflect spring qualities: cool, stable, moist, and heavy. They have a strong, dense structure, but with a low metabolism, they can easily put on weight. Like springtime, they retain water and tend to accumulate mucous. Therefore, a lifestyle that allows a natural bodily water and energy flow is essential to weight management. They have a steady, but moderate appetite, and can easily miss a meal. They are slower moving and generally resist exercise.

Emotionally, *Kapha* are the same traits as the physical: earthy, solid, stable, grounded, sensual, and steady personality that can handle changes and stress well overall. When balanced, they are calm, dependable peacekeepers, cool tempered and affectionate. When out of balance, they are depressed, sluggish, congested, and overweight. They need to especially care for their lymphatic system, lungs, and stomach.

The Kapha body type should consume more light grains, proteins, vegetables, and heating and pungent spices for their warming properties to offset this cooler type. They should eat less heavy, fatty proteins, dairy, gluten-based grains, and starchy vegetables. The spring body type should include plenty of cleansing foods for good elimination, such as leafy greens, sprouts, berries, and some citrus fruits.

After the spring heaviness, we come to the summer heat, the Pitta body type, having a medium body frame, a moderate weight, and good musculature. The Pitta dosha elements are *fire and water.* The Pitta reflects the summer qualities: hot, humid, (perspiring) sharp, and penetrating. They carry a well-proportioned body, prone to muscularity, but easily overheated. Like the Pitta time of day, they have a strong metabolism and need to eat regularly. They may also be vulnerable to skin rashes and infections.

Emotionally, the Pitta mirrors similar characteristics: a Type A personality, laser focused, compelled to accomplish tasks, productive, organized, and energetic. Like the physical strong digestion, Pittas have a robust, mental digestive quality to perceive and assimilate reality. Like the summer needs rain for cooling, so the Pitta needs a *cooling* lifestyle. When balanced, Pitta's are courageous, competitive, capable, and clear communicators with creative problem solving skills. When out of balance, they may have heated reactions such as anger or jealously.

The Pitta body type should consume more cooling foods such as fruits, melons, vegetables, sweet and bitter spices, and adequate proteins for endurance, reducing spicy, heating foods and drinks. They should nourish the eyes, small intestine, blood, spleen, gall bladder, and liver.

As the summer heat is gradually brushed away with colder temperatures, *Vata* appears. Like the winter trees show their bare, slender twigs, so this body type has a thin, delicate bone structure, is slim, and light weight. The Vata dosha element is air, reflecting airy qualities: sensitive, spiritual, perceptive, and can quickly move, speak, and think, like an ice skater gracefully gliding through midair. Their digestive pattern can be irregular, like winter hibernation, and they may have dry *winter* skin.

Emotionally, Vatas portray the winter qualities: like camouflaged snowy scenery, they may be creative, with propensity toward arts, or abstract thinkers. When balanced, they tend to be mentally sharp and quick, expressive, enthusiastic, and energetic. When out of balance, they can easily become overwhelmed, flighty, and anxious, lose weight, become constipated, and have weakened immunity and an unsteady nervous system. They may have sleep and nervous challenges. The *Vata* especially needs a balanced structure to stay on course, such as adequate sleep, warming foods to offset coldness, and stress releasing exercise.

The *Vata* body type needs to care for the nervous system,

colon, and bones. Increase warming, lubricating, grounding, heavier foods such as stews, nuts, grains, and warming proteins, and decrease raw and cold foods and low-fat diets.

Our distinct body type is part of our divine design carrying us through our destination. As we understand our own unique body type, we can appreciate and nourish ourselves with a lifestyle that supports our strengths and weaknesses.

Health Coach Recommendations

- Like spring, Kapha tends to retain water and needs open pathways to release toxins and excess water, with plenty of cleansing foods. Emotionally, the same is true. They tend to hold on to toxic emotions and can become lethargic, dull, depressed, and overweight. This strong body type needs aerobic and cardiovascular exercise to maintain a healthy flow. Self-acceptance body-image affirmations will help Kapha love their body; like a horse will never have the body type of a deer, yet it's is admired for its amazing strength, endurance, and beauty.
- As summer temperatures soar, Pitta's are hot and need to chill out to prevent overheating with cooling drinks like peppermint tea and refreshing limes, melons, and grapes. This *ever-ready battery* also needs to keep charged with summer's array of fiberous, sustainable vegetables and fruits, accompanied by proteins. When the heat soars emotionally, Pittas need to vent the heat in a healthy way. Calming and relaxing exercise, activities, and meditations helps keep this driven body type on the right road.
- Then winter undresses the trees, and the cold wind causes dryness. Like the thin, but acrobatic squirrels who confidently leap through space and find nuts (natural oils, protein, and nutrition) to insolate and sustain through the harsh winter, so Vatas thrive on *comfort foods* such as warm cooked soups, stews, starchy and root vegetables, grains, and protein. Vatas can help prevent the tendency for worry and anxiety and

promote appropriate weight by maintaining a balanced lifestyle with adequate sleep, warm moist foods, physical warmth, and tension-relieving activities like yoga, pilates, and weight bearing exercise to build stamina. While this type may feel distant and forgetful, they have an astounding capacity to leap for success in academics and arts.

Recommended Readings:

Ayurveda: A Life of Balance: The Complete Guide to Ayurvedic Nutrition & Body Types with Recipes by Maya Tiwari
Textbook of Ayurveda, Vol. 1: Fundamental Principles of Ayurveda 1st Edition by Vasant Lad

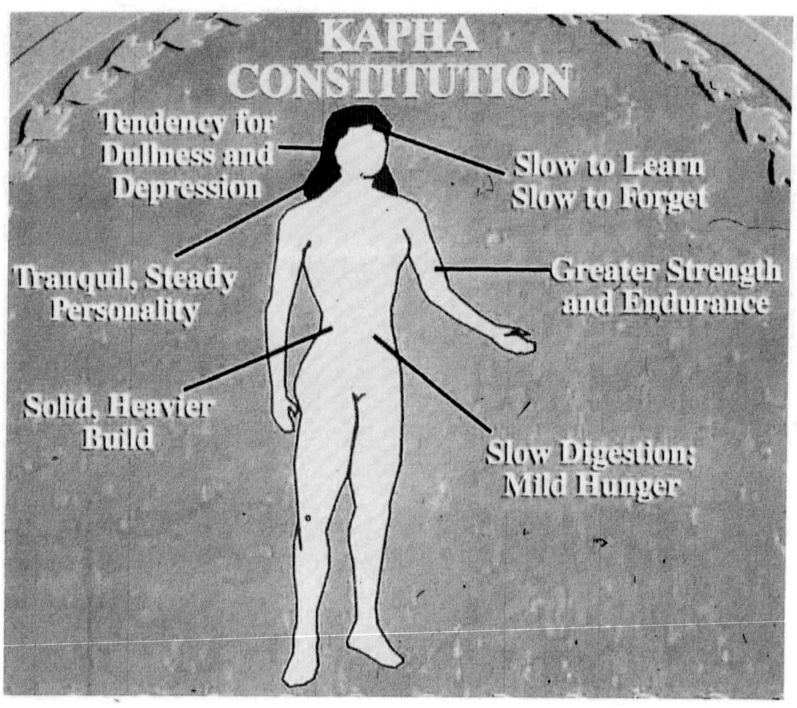

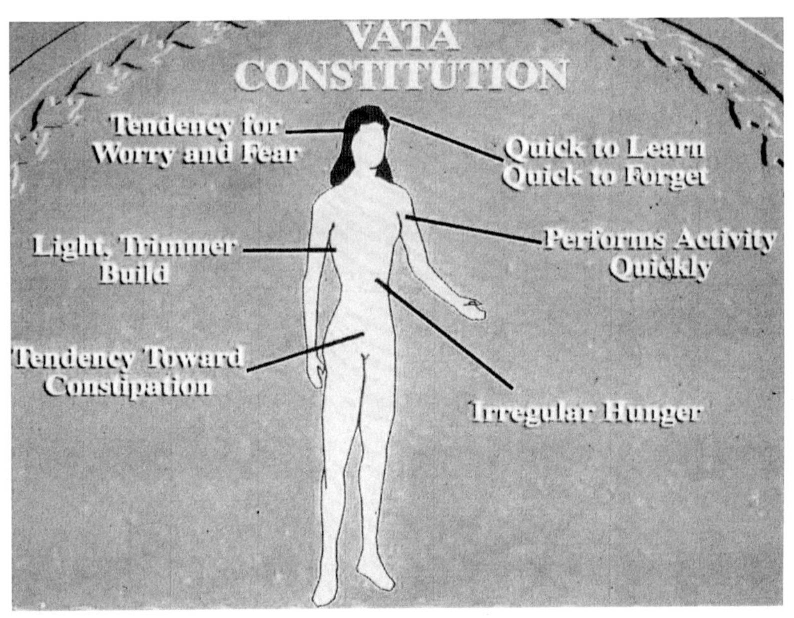
VATA
CONSTITUTION
Tendency for
Worry and Fear
Quick to Learn
Quick to Forget
Light, Trimmer
Build
Performs Activity
Quickly
Tendency Toward
Constipation
Irregular Hunger

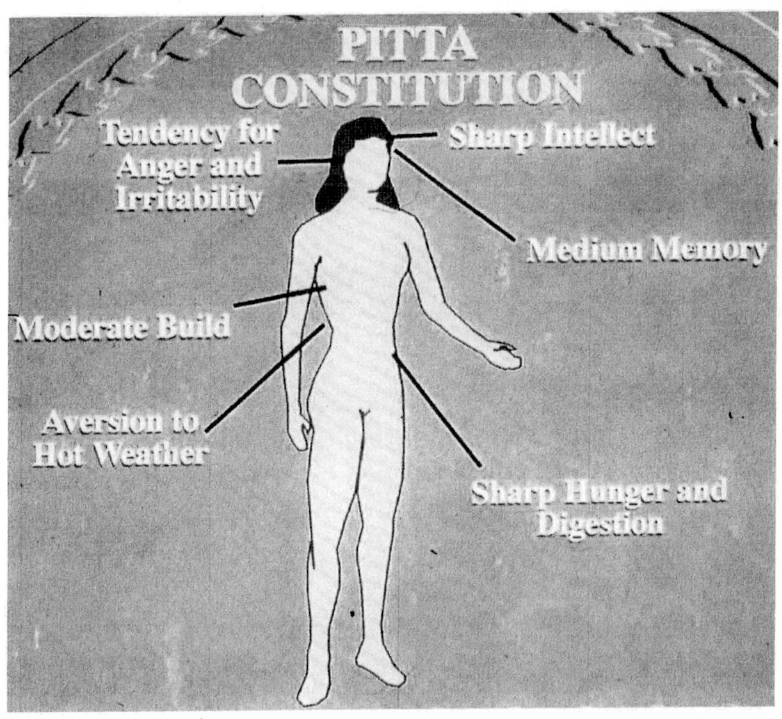
PITTA
CONSTITUTION
Tendency for
Anger and
Irritability
Sharp Intellect
Medium Memory
Moderate Build
Aversion to
Hot Weather
Sharp Hunger and
Digestion

In the Ayurvedic science, body types are determined by size, which then projects the ideal self-care for each individual. As for physical exercise, body type is also distinguished by shape, which guides us to sculpting our vessels to the glory of the Lord. This artful science of physical fitness was well developed by Dr. Joseph Christiano, a renowned physical fitness trainer and naturopathy doctor who teaches how physical fitness links to godliness:

When you dedicate the entire process to God, your body will become a temple of honor, filled with his presence. (*My Body, My Temple*, 36)

Your Fruit Shape

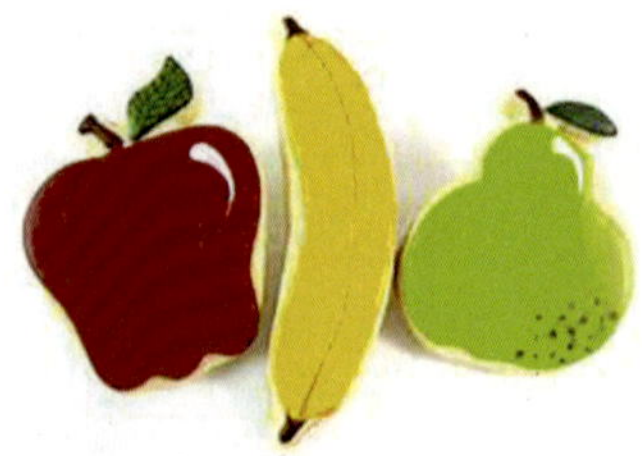

Consider how the condition and appearance of your physical body glorifies God. While the Lord is primarily concerned with the heart of man, think of the Lord's specific instructions for the cosmetic beauty in building the tabernacle. How much more passionate He must be about the vitality of His living temple – You?! What a testimony of God's best – a healthy robust body infused by His divine seed. How pleasing it must be to the Lord as we sculpt his masterpiece.

Does the shape of your body resemble an *apple, banana,* or *pear?* The answer to this will help you prepare an exercise routine that maintains body weight in proper proportion. You can determine your shape by anwering this question: When you put on weight, where does most of the weight go? If on the lower body (hips, buttocks, and thighs), you would be the *pear.* If on the upper body (chest, back, tummy, and arms), you would be the *apple.* If on the upper and lower body (all of the above), you would be a banana.

Once you define your fruit shape, you can begin your divine makeover. This fitness program is tailored to enhance your genetic structure, synchronizing the whole body. The directives for each body shape is below. The complete exercise program is given in the appendix of Dr. Joseph Christiano's book, *Blood types, Body types and YOU.*

The *pear* shape distributes weight in the lower body, while the upper body is usually smaller, with a shallow bustline and narrow shoulders. The pear shape can be redesigned by broadening the chest/bust, arms, and shoulders and building muscle mass, while toning and lengthening the lower half.

The *apple* shape accumulates weight in the upper body, while the lower body is generally thinner, with slender legs by the buttocks. The apple shape is remodeled by strengthening the upper and lower legs and by building muscle mass while toning and lengthening the upper half.

The *banana* shape disperses weight equally in the upper and lower body, forming a straight line, without shapeliness. The banana is reformed by firming and toning the abdominal muscles to create some curvature between the upper and lower half while lengthening and strengthening the thighs and buttocks.

As you see, knowing your types allows you to design a self care package that unwraps optimal health. Your seasonal body type and emotional type portrays a comprehensive healthy lifestyle encompassing general exercise, diet, and emotional well-being. Your blood type dictates specific foods that are highly beneficial and those to avoid. Your body shape determines a body-sculpting program to enhance your natural features and compensate for imbalance. Rather than adopting a cookie cutter program that fits someone else, this enables you to instinctively eat and live according to your genetic base and sculpt your body in a way that is symetrically pleasing, making you feel your best, honoring the Lord and yourself –U-nique beautiful You!

Spiritual Reflection of Seasons

And let us not grow weary of doing good, for in due season we will reap, if we do not give up (Gal. 6:9 ESV).

We have seen how the annual seasons are paralleled in the daily cycles, reflecting the seasons in each day. Now consider a Genesis perspective.

First, let's see the numerical significance of numbers which reflect the age of Moses, Abraham, (and Sarah) as presented by Dr. Ibojie in *The Illustrated Significance of Dream Symbols:*

70: Universality or restoration. The Israelites lived in exile for **70** years and were restored **70** years later.

80: Beginning of a high calling...Moses was **80** years old when he started his ministry to deliver the Israelites.

90 or **99:** Fruits are ripe and ready. Abraham *"was ninety years and nine when God appeared to him"* (Gen. 17:1)

100: God's election of grace, full reward, or children of promise. *"Abraham was a hundred years old when his son Isaac was born to him"* (Gen. 21:5)

Most of the great ideas, inventions, and masterpieces throughout history were performed by those who were over 50! Fifty, according to Ibojie, is the number for the Holy Spirit, which was poured out 50 days after Christ's resurrection. As you see, from the Genesis perspective, we truly ripen richly as we age.

Yet, we tend to see the seasons in our *lifetime* in a limited, shallow way. For instance, we might envision our first 25 years as our blossoming springtime; then the next 25 years as our productive summer, and finally, the last years as our barren winter.

But God has a different viewpoint from His aerial view. Over the course of time, the *Master Potter* is ultimately molding us into the shape of Jesus, to become as He is… in His image.

During our spring and summer, the Holy Spirit cultivates and tills our rocky soil, restores our eroding banks, weeds out the toxic residue, blows away the chaff, and plants seeds of faith that will flourish in full bloom in the *harvest* season.

He exhorts us not to grow weary during our cultivating time as we faithfully do the good work that He implores us to do, though we still may not see a sprout. Sometimes the Lord is preparing our circumstances (positioning relationships, events, changes, etc.) and other times He is preparing us to receive the fullness of His blessing. In fact, we may not see or accept the blessing in our pre-mature season. Yet, as we trust our heavenly Father to turn our rocky clay into a rich, fertile ground, we will reap the harvest, perhaps just when we thought we were losing ground. May we be inspired by many who, in their fabulous fifties or beyond, reaped their bountiful harvest, like these contemporary examples:

- Ronald Regan wasn't elected to his first public office until he was 55 years old.
- Alexander Graham Bell perfected the telephone at 58 and resolved the stabilization of airplanes in his 70's.
- George Burns won his first Oscar at 80.
- Colonel Sanders began his famous Kentucky Fried Chicken at 65.
- Michelangelo painted the Sistine Chapel at 71.
- Golda Meir became Prime Minister of Israel at 71.
- Grandma Moses began painting at 78 (with arthritis), and by 88, she was a world renowned artist with pictures in galleries worldwide when she was age 90. At 100, birthday greetings came in from around the world. In 1961, she passed away at 101.

Over 60% of the world's greatest work has been achieved by people over 60!

"Your mind is still young at 50 – your brain doesn't reach its zenith until 10 years after that. And from 60 on, mental efficiency declines very slowly to the age of 80. At 80, you can be just as productive mentally as you were at 30 – and you should know a lot more"; Dr. George Lawson, a gerontologist, cited in *First Thing Every Morning* by Timberlake Lewis, p. 80

Who satisfies your years with good things, So that your youth is renewed like the eagle (Psalm 103:5 NASB).

From man's peephole view, it may be all downhill after forty, but from the Lord's heavenly view, we are soaring on eagle's wings until the day we fly home to Him. Until then, He has given us many health and healing modalities to finish strong with a bountiful harvest.

In the final chapter of this section, we'll explore yet two more ways to preserve our youthfulness, reducing stress in body and mind, with two Genesis gems.

The clues for uncovering these *gemstones: Adam and Eve* and the *breath of life.*

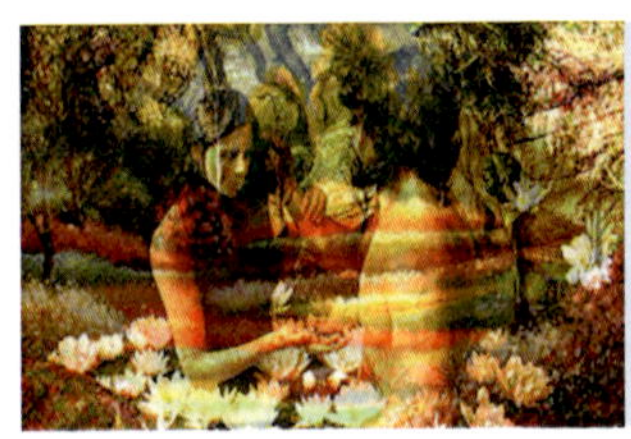

Chapter 9

Nourishing the Physical and Emotional body

Then the LORD God made a woman from the rib he had taken out of the man, and he brought her to the man (Gen. 2:22).

Isn't it amazing how God took this small *piece* of man, to fulfill man's missing *piece*? Likewise, women are fulfilled, as they age, by a small *piece* of man - It's *testosterone*!

What does this male hormone have to do with women? Everything. Testosterone greatly acelerates healing and is the foundation for building and maintaining muscle, bone, energy, and libido. Without adequate levels of testosterone, a woman can't build muscle adequately. We see the crucial role of this hormone, considering that the heart is also a muscle. It not only brings a woman to life, but preserves her life. Ironically, the *bone* from which a woman was created is the one that sustains her own bones. Furthermore, it promotes balance, preventing falls, which are quite common in elderly women without sufficient testosterone levels. It even makes a woman *feel* more *womanly*.

As for men, what happens when testosterone slowly seeps away? Everything - times 10! Since men need about ten times as much as women, sufficient levels provide all of these benefits, to a greater degree. It increases confidence, stamina in all ways, and helps protect from mentally declining disease, cancer, etc.

While the recommendations and healing modalities covered thus far promote a healthy lifestyle, we are best conditioned by replenishing that which erodes in the aging process. This is where bio-identical (all natural) hormone replacement comes to the rescue. It is the exact replica of the human hormone, without a host of possible side effects.

Hormones work in concert together within a delicate balance, back to Adam and Eve. Hormonal balance is perhaps one of the most vital, but misunderstood, elements of maintaining optimal health, for both men and women. Since this is complex, here we'll only attempt to highlight some of the benefits of natural hormone replacements and the effects of deficiencies.

Hormone levels gradually begin declining in the mid to late 30's. In the 40's, it's common to have symptoms related to thyroid hormone deficiency, and in the 50's, it's *uncommon* to have an optimally functioning thyroid. When the thyroid isn't properly functioning, often one's weight increases and energy levels decrease, among many other symptoms. According to Dr. Frank Shallenberger, in his book, *Bursting with Energy,* 231, "*All the other hormones are dependent on the thyroid gland for their optimal functioning.*"

A hormone specialist orders extensive lab tests to prepare the precise levels for each individual. This customized perscription is prepared by a compound pharmacy, usually in the form of creams and capsules (and can be purchased inexpensively). Furthermore, this delicate web of hormone replacements is monitored for possible adjustments.

Dr. Shallenberger further explains that synthetic hormones are prescribed because they are often more profitable. *A naturally occurring substance is not patenable, such as bio-identical hormone replacements. Synthetic hormones are not really hormones at all, they are drugs with hormone-like effects. One of the common ones, for example, is made from horses. It's a hormone replacement for a horse, but a drug for humans.* Is it any wonder why one might have severe side effects?

Yet, the rejuvenating effects of bio-identical hormone replacements are wonderful! Dr. Shallenberger shares some of these benefits:

- Better mood and sleep
- Built-in resistence to illness and infections

- Enhanced healing
- Enhanced sexual performance
- Fat loss without dieting
- Fortified brain, heart, kidneys, liver, spleen, and other organs that atrophy with aging
- Improved cardiac function
- Increased exercise capacity
- Increased muscle mass without exercising
- Lower blood presure
- Lower LDL cholesterol, the bad cholesterol that contributes to harmful plaque
- Reduced wrinkles and tighter, thicker skin
- Strengthened bones
- Youthful energy production

Some patients, says Dr. Shallenberger, ask if natural hormone therapy is safe. With a benefits package like this and no harmful side effects, he responds with the flip side of this question: Is it *safe not* to replenish hormones as needed? In the same way, is it safe not to take necessary medicines, supplements, or whatever you need for optimal health?

Personally, my family's experience with natural hormone therapy has been most profound. About two months after my 80 year old mother began therapy, her spinal bone density test showed a 50% improvement! After my husband started therapy, he became more muscular and noticed accelerated healing in his knee injury. As for myself, I stopped waking throughout the night and finally slept much better, improving my energy level.

Spiritual Reflection of Adam and Eve

So God created mankind in his own image, in the image of God he created them; male and female he created them (Gen. 1:27).

We discussed how polar opposites create balance and harmony in the other elements of creation, such as light, colors, and seasons.

Finally, Adam and Eve are the most amazing polar opposites, the pinnacle of creation, with a triple emphasis on created in His image. How beautifully these polar opposites create balance in each other!

How do these *physical* gender attributes reflect the spirit of God? Let us consider the qualities of a man and a woman, expressing the sacred beauty of Our Creator.

The physical nature of man is strong, bulky, and firm, like the ground from which he came, while the physical nature of a woman is generally delicate, smaller, and pliable, like the rib from which she came. Men are usually more aggressive and external, while women are generally more subtle and *internal* (again, like the rib). In fact, women can be so subtle that all of those little hints and clues just fly right over her man! Yet, we can learn how the strengths of both genders are *fused together* in the mighty works of the Lord, played out in a symphony of *logic* and *emotion* through many biblical stories.

One of my favorites is when Nathan the prophet confronts King David about his affair with Bathsheba. The prophet shares a very *subtle* story with the king that stirs up the king's aggressive emotions. Then Nathan lands a powerful punch – the story about a little lamb that causes the King to repent. Similarly, when Jesus defended the woman in adultery, He subtly roused emotions with an indisputable confrontation leaving the accusers speechless.

Many times, the Lord forcefully fought for His people, parting the seas, and striking the enemy. Other times, He quietly escorted people or circumstances *undercover* to accomplish Divine purposes, such as Mary and Joseph's secret departure.

At times, we see the Lord's firm position towards man's misdeeds in the form of consequences, while in other cases softer, as when Abraham negotiated with God regarding the destruction of a city if only a few righteous men were there. Similarly in our own lives, we can see these two forms of divine energy at work: the powerful arm of the Lord strengthening and defending us, while the compassionate hand of the Lord touches us with tender mercies.

These dual genders are also mirrored in all of nature. Strong stable tree trunks support curvy limbs that are laden with intricate dangling leaves, and are rivaled by fragrant blossoms and tempting fruits. The ocean thrashes and roars with powerful waves and sweeping currents, winding down into gentle lapping waves. Likewise, the sun piercingly penetrates all of life, giving way to the mystical softer light - the moon, a gentle power that silently, but powerfully, controls the sea tides! Indeed, the earth in all of its majesty and mystery proclaims the glory of the Lord! *"O Lord, how manifold are your works! In wisdom you have made them after all"* (Psalm 104:24 NIV).

Finally, the dual genders are expressed in Christ's relationship to the Church – His Bride. With Christ as the divine Groom, the two seamlessly merge as one. Christ supports and protects his Church, for he is the root and *trunk* of her life. She is the maturing and blossoming Bride who reaches out with compassionate hands to nurture the world. Herein is the great mystery unfolded – that we would be as He is — realizing our complete potential in his likeness, fully expressing the totality of God by the artful dance of the dual genders. We truly are the magnificence of His handiwork.

Emotional Wellness

When treading through the deep waters of emotions, it is only the Holy Spirit who can separate the thoughts from the intents of the heart, and seeking His guidance truly fulfills our destiny.

Since emotions all flow together, it can be difficult to recognize and distinguish our various emotional needs. Yet, our emotional well-being certainly deserves the same attention, if not more, than our physical.

Consider these five emotional needs that easily overlap, but each contributes significantly to wellness. For each individual, this is a personal decision, and of course, everyone's circumstances determine what's right and best. Therefore, the first step is acknowledging these emotional needs in our natural design: 1) love, 2) friendship, 3) touch, 4) intimacy, and 5) sex (according to one's proper relationship).

For instance, in a marital relationship, this might provide a forum to understand the mutual needs and encourage communication. For an individual, this can be a place of meditation and prayer in seeking the Lord's guidance. By recognizing and fulfilling each need (again, in accordance to one's proper relationship), we begin to feel *fully alive*!

In conclusion of nourishing the physical and emotional body, this greatest gem of creation, Adam and Eve reflecting the image of God, merits wholehearted attention. We were designed to enjoy all of these emotional outlets even as we age. This is where natural hormone replacement can help keep the marital bed a sweet *Garden of Eden*.

The Breath of Life

Then the LORD God formed a man from the dust of the ground and breathed into his nostrils the breath of life, and the man became a living being (Gen. 2:7).

God breathed in man the breath of life. In this way, *breath, life, and energy* are all equivalent, and by increasing one, you are increasing the others. Therefore, we can preserve our energy and longevity, especially by sustaining pure, active oxygen, in the air we breathe and in our food and drink.

Since plants are our oxygen source, imagine the quality of air in the Garden of Eden. Scientists were able to analyze air bubbles trapped in 80 million year old amber and discovered that the oxygen level was more than 30%! (No wonder the dinosaurs were huge.) The average oxygen level today is about 21%. Some highly polluted areas measure only about 10%, and the minimum level for existence is 7%. We evolved from an oxygen rich environment that far supersedes our present oxygen lifestyle. Therefore, our focus should be on upgrading our oxygen quality, internally, externally, and maximizing our reception.

We generally think of oxygen as only external, the air we breathe into our lungs. Yet this is only the beginning. It is the oxygen that is actually delivered at the cellular level that makes us thrive. As green plants provide oxygen externally, so they do for us internally when we consume them.

Recall back in chapter two that Dr. Miley made the milestone discovery that blood irradiation actually *oxygenates* the blood, which is why this method was such an effective antibiotic treatment. Indeed, oxygen is the body's primary way of cleansing itself. When toxins are bound with oxygen, the bodily systems can escort them out, rather than becoming stagnant.

According to Ed McCabe, "Mr. Oxygen," "… the vast majority of disease causing microbes absolutely cannot live in active forms of oxygen! Almost every virus, bacteria, fungi, microplasm, parasite, and other pathogen found in all diseases including HIV, arthritis, heart disease, cancer, chronic fatigue…and every other disease… all have the same…life forms…anaerobic. The disease bugs simply can't live in *active* oxygen."(p. 57)

In his book, *Flood Your Body with Oxygen*, Ed McCabe explains that this is the key to warding off disease and sickness and creating a wellspring of energy. He shares many types of *oxygen therapies* to flood your body with oxygen for optimum health.

Another significant aspect of increasing energy and relieving stress is our ability to take in oxygen efficiently. Proper breathing increases your oxygen intake into the lungs, and released in the cells, leads to greater energy production with less tension and anxiety, among other benefits. It also contributes *aerobic* energy production (energy produced from oxygen), rather than *anaerobic* (energy produced without oxygen).

Breathing techiniques also fortify us with oxygen. According to Dr. Shallenberger, *Abdominal breathing* increases *aerobic* energy, while *chest-wall breathing* uses *anaerobic energy*.

Think about how you breathe during an emergency. Your breathing usually becomes short and shallow, with both the chest-wall and abdomen rapidly pulsating. This momentary change in breathing maximizes energy to respond to the crisis. After the alarming situation, we might feel exhausted from the excess *energy sprint*. As our circumstances return to normal, so should our breathing, ideally back to abdominal breathing.

If however, you experience chronic stress or anxiety, your breathing might stay in chest-wall breathing mode, causing lingering fatigue. This type of breathing requires about twice as many breaths per minute than does abdominal breathing. Chest-wall breathers work double-time to get the same oxygen. Additionally, the excess loss of carbon dioxide changes the PH balance of the blood, leading to anxiety and stress. It can also increase muscular tension in the shoulder area. Therefore, abdominal breathing is more efficient and increases energy production.

Abdominal breathing is when your abdomen moves as you breathe, and your chest remains still. This is the diaphragmatic breathing technique that singers learn to retain enough oxygen for a smooth voice. Instructions for this more efficient breathing pattern are provided by Dr. Frank Shallenberger in *Bursting With Energy*, "Breathing Right."

Aerobic oxygen is also greatly increased by *aerobic exercise*. Even though oxygen levels may be normal in the body, adequate oxygen doesn't completely *penetrate to the cells* without aerobic exercise. *Moderate* aerobic exercise is the key. It brings us to an aerobic level without overly exerting into the *anaerobic*-threshold, which reverses to energy supplied without adequate oxygen. This point of *overdrive* actually becomes unhealthy, increasing free-radicals, with more vulnerability to disease and injury. Furthermore, it is counterproductive to weight loss, causing stress hormones to *lock in* fat in response to stress. Instructions for balanced, efficient exercise are also given in *Bursting With Energy*, "Exercise."

Furthermore, *Nasal* breathing versus *mouth* breathing is a optimal way of taking in the *breath of life*. During exercise, breathing in through the nose allows air to flow deeply into the lower lobes of the lungs to disperse throughout the body. Nasal breathing has many benefits, such as better circulation, increased blood oxygen, stabilized carbon dioxide levels, regulates the breathing rate, kills bacteria, creates an internal air conditioning, and minimizes the chances of catching flies in the mouth (just kidding). Mouth breathing creates a *false alarm* that carbon dioxide is escaping the body too quickly, which stimulates mucous production, and the body then attempts to slow the breathing.

Finally, nasal breathing techniques are effective stress busters. Here's a simple one you can do at any moment. Slowly inhale through your nose for a count of eight, briefly pause, and slowly exhale through your mouth for a count of eight, briefly pause, and repeat three to four times.

Spiritual Reflection of Breath

During the night, a powerful gusty storm blew across our lawn. When we awoke, the neighbor's trampoline had not only blown over a tall fence and into our yard, but it somehow landed on *its feet*. Ironically, the trampoline itself had done an acrobatic *flip*, landing perfectly upright. On the front lawn, the storm took down large branches of an old, deceasing tree.

This is how the breath of God blows in our lives, often during our *nights*, and when we are *sleeping* in those dormant times when we can do *nothing* but trust Him to do *everything*. That's when the mighty wind moves us in into places or positions that we never dreamed of, like a whirlwind that lands us directly *on our feet* in the president's office, or in the presence of our soulmate. On the other side, The Lord is blowing away the branches of our deceasing *old man*, as we are becoming more like Him, a new creation!

"Then the channels of water appeared, and the foundations of the world were laid bare At Your rebuke, O LORD, at the blast of the breath of Your nostrils" (Psalms 18:15 ESV).

Jesus further expounds on this analogy as he teaches Nicodemus (and all who have ears to hear).

"The wind blows wherever it pleases. You hear its sound, but you cannot tell where it comes from or where it is going. So it is with everyone born of the Spirit" (John 3:8).

What an amazing blessing to be born of the Spirit, surrendering the helm of our life's sails to the Lord, and being blown along a voyage that leads to His destinations!

He personally demonstrates this to his disciples, with a beautiful parallel to our creation. As God breathed life into our physical being, so the Lord breathed life into our spirit being.

So Jesus said to them again, *"Peace be with you; as the Father has sent Me, I also send you." And when He had said this, He breathed on them and said to them, "Receive the Holy Spirit"* (John 20:21-22).

Our new birth is only the beginning of the *breathtaking* breath of God. He yearns to breathe life into every crevice of our life. God breathed His word, which becomes our living breath, the spiritual *oxygen* that becomes the energy of our lives.

Joel Osteen reminds his listeners that the winds of God's favor are shifting our lives in new directions to receive healing, fresh opportunities and new breakthroughs.

"The greatest force in the universe is breathing your way—it's the favor of Almighty God. God can cause the winds of favor to blow opportunity, healing, and breakthroughs into your life. Suddenly, one touch from Him can shift you from sickness to health, lack to abundance, struggle to ease. Doors that did not open before will suddenly open. What should have taken years, with God's touch, can happen in a fraction of the time. God has unlimited ways to turn any situation around! All we have to do is believe" (Joel Osteen, *Break Out).*

Indeed, the wind of the Holy Spirit is blowing amazing blessings into the life that we live now. I always find it refreshing to be reminded that eternity includes now! Furthermore, as we *breathe in* the Spirit deeply by our prayers, in worship, the Lord escorts us to the deep caverns of *His* breath, overflowing with joy, goodness, peace, and *longsuffering*. Who knew more about *longsuffering* than Job?

In the book of Job, we find many references to the breath of God, perhaps an indication of Job's intimate relationship with God. And what could be more intimate than the breath of God?

"The Spirit of God has made me, And the breath of the Almighty gives me life" (Job 33:4 NLT).

"But it is a spirit in man, And the breath of the Almighty gives them understanding" (Job 32:8 NASB).

"By His breath the heavens are cleared; His hand has pierced the fleeing serpent" (Job 26:13 NASB).

"By the breath of God they perish, And by the blast of His anger they come to an end" (Job 4:9 NASB).

As we see, Job was a man who knew the breath of God, and intimately breathed in the Lord, thereby sustaining the unimaginable and received a double portion after his losses. Both the language and lessons of Job provide profound insight for divine healing, which bridges us into the final section of *The Gems of Genesis.* Note that Job calls his enemy *the fleeing serpent.* Also, even though Job is distraught and in great pain, he doesn't surrender to his miserable comforter's *blame game.*

The final scripture that links the breath of God to divine healing is so astounding that it must close the curtains of this section and make a grand opening for the next chapter:

Again He said to me, "Prophesy over these bones and say to them, 'O dry bones, hear the word of the LORD.' Thus says the Lord GOD to these bones, 'Behold, I will cause breath to enter you that you may come to life. I will put sinews on you, make flesh grow back on you, cover you with skin and put breath in you that you may come alive; and you will know that I am the Lord'" (Ezekiel 37:4-6 NASB).

Breathe on me, breath of God,
Fill me with life anew,
That I may love what Thou dost love,
And do what Thou wouldst do.

Breathe on me, breath of God,
Until my heart is pure,
Until with Thee I will one will,
To do and to endure.

Breathe on me, breath of God,
Blend all my soul with Thine,
Until this earthly part of me
Glows with Thy fire divine.

Breathe on me, breath of God,
So shall I never die,
But live with Thee the perfect life
Of Thine eternity.

Health Coach Recommendations

- After 40, seek counsel from a hormone specialist who can check all hormonal levels. A directory can be found on American Academy of Anti-Aging Medicine at www.world-health.net, or call 773-528-1000.
- Use the deep breathing exercise for an immedite stress buster.
- Breath meditations can help you relax and unwind.
- Consider all of your emotional needs and how they are a part of optimal health.

Recommended Readings:

Flood Your Body with Oxygen by Ed McCabe
The Testosterone Syndrome by Eugene Shippen, MD & William Fryer
Bursting with Energy by Frank Shallenberger, MD, HMD

Part 3

Spiritual Nutrition

(divine design)

Having surveyed the cornerstones of health in the physical elements of creation, i.e. night, sunlight, rainbow light, seasons, land and water, plants and animals, and finally, Adam and Eve, we now consider the spiritual elements of our *new creation,* our divine design – the image of God.

The many healing modalities in the physical realm emanating from creation makes it quite evident that God yearns for health and healing in our lives. Yet, how to grasp this through faith, may at times feel unattainable. As we are spiritually nourished, we can receive complete healing of every health condition or disease.

Divine healing may occur immediately, in a miraculous way, or in the process of time, as the gifts of healing. By merging both the scientific laws in the natural, and the spiritual laws in the supernatural, we release the power of God in amazing ways. When we use tangible means as a bridge to the intangible, we enter a place where all things are possible.

The Law of Attraction teaches concrete ways to increase our expectation, thereby building our faith. The Law of Restoration exemplifies the eight P's of healing restoration: perspective, promise, passion, persistence, patience, positioning, presence, and performance. The Law of Fulfillment demonstrates how fulfilling our values is the core of our well-being.

Finally, we nourish our spirit by fulfilling our divine purpose, as we receive our healing, and assist others in healing too. These principles all work together for health and fulfillment as beautifully portrayed by our Genesis fathers, each in their own unique way.

Principles of Divine Healing

When faith comes to our spirit, as naturally as seeing and hearing comes to our body, we will speak the breath of life into our mortal bodies that we may glorify God.

Again He said to me, "Prophesy over these bones and say to them, 'O dry bones, hear the word of the LORD.' "Thus says the Lord GOD to these bones, 'Behold, I will cause breath to enter you that you may come to life. 'I will put sinews on you, make flesh grow back on you, cover you with skin and put breath in you that you may come alive; and you will know that I am the Lord" (Ezekiel 37:4-14 NASB).

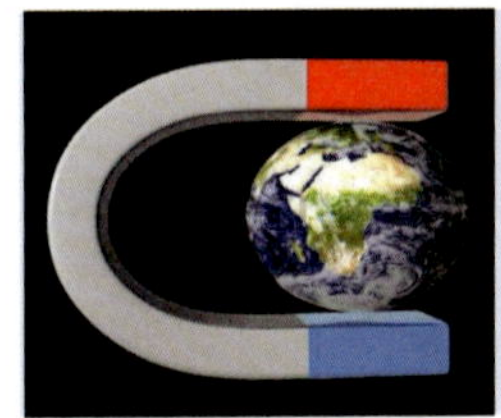

Chapter 10
The Law of Attraction

And He brought him forth abroad and said, "Look now toward heaven, and count the stars, if thou be able to count them"; and He said unto him, "So shall thy seed be" (Genesis 15:5 JSP).

But you promised me, *"I will surely treat you kindly, and I will multiply your descendants until they become as numerous as the sands along the seashore — too many to count"* (Genesis 32:12 NLT).

Notice that along with God's *promise* of abundance, he also creates a *picture* of abundance for Abraham. During the day, as Abraham treaded across the desert terrain, he saw grains of sand, the symbol of his inheritance, and God's promise was being *ingrained* in his mind. Perhaps, pondering all of this, he might have picked up a handful of sand and watched the innumerable grains trickle through the crevice of his fingers. In the night, the stars were constantly before him, glowing through the evening backdrop of the sky even as he slept. Thus, these two abiding images, the sand and the stars, became the *screensavers* of his mind.

Not only did God provide dominant *images*, but also a powerful *word*. Not just a word, but Abraham's own name took on a new meaning. The magnetic force of faith, through images and words, enabled him to remain steadfast against all of the evidence of nature that said, "No way!" Every time Abraham said his new name, he was affirming the promise *verbally*, while the sand and stars were confirming the promise *visually*.

No longer will you be called Abram; your name will be Abraham, for I have made you a father of many nations (Genesis 17:5).

The Lord used these tangible elements to help him anchor the intangible; stars in the night — sand in the day, a continual reminder of God's faithfulness.

Likewise, Jacob utilized this principle of focus, but in a unique way, with the livestock presently belonging to Laban, his father-in-law. Jacob's observant endeavor with sheep breeding would eventually pay him dividends as he bargained to get the best animals from his father-in-law. Jacob peeled back the tree bark, exposing the speckled interior, and as the sheep mated with this image continually before them, *the flocks brought forth striped, speckled, and spotted [sheep]...* a premium breed!

Then Jacob took fresh rods of poplar and almond and plane trees, and peeled white stripes in them, exposing the white which was in the rods. He set the rods which he had peeled in front of the flocks in the gutters, even in the watering troughs, where the flocks came to drink; and they mated when they came to drink. So the flocks mated by the rods, and the flocks brought forth striped, speckled, and spotted... (Genesis 30: 37–39 NASB).

Here in Genesis are wonderful examples of what we know today as the science of the Law of Attraction. In recent years, Michael J. Losier, in his book, *The Law of Attraction,* has developed this into a step-by-step application used to help individuals and businesses prosper in any area they seek. In this chapter, we'll see how we can utilize these simple, powerful tools to glorify God in our own health and prosperity.

Beloved, I pray that in all respects you may prosper and be in good health, just as your soul prospers (3 John 1:2 NASB).

Faith can only rise as high as our images and words. Let us now learn how to raise the *vibration* of our images and words.

What is the Law of Attraction, and how does it work?

The vibrational world is the powerful undercurrent of the universe. As we have seen how vibrations are the healing power of light therapy, so this is the underlying effect of other healing arts, such as sound therapy. It is the *energy of vibrations* that also governs the *Law of Attraction (L.O. A.), since vibrations* control the most basic polar opposites, *negative* and *positive.*

The L.O.A. was first known, ironically, as the *Teachings of Abraham*, as introduced and taught by Esther and Jerry Hicks. Since then, these profound concepts have been taught in workshops and seminars around the world, propelling success in individuals and businesses in every arena of life. The L.O.A. is powerful because it builds a framework for faith in practical application.

Michael J. Losier has developed a step-by-step powerful series to attain goals and desires for both corporate and personal use. He describes the Law of Attraction (L.O. A.) as "*the science of attracting more of what you want and less of what you don't.*" He defines it as *"I attract to my life whatever I give my attention, focus, and energy to, whether positive or negative."*(p.12)

Our minds are truly magnets. They rapidly accumulate *more of the same.* As a small fistful of snow descends down a white snowy hill, it becomes a large *white globe* at the foot of the hill. Similarly, when a snowball rolls down a *muddy* snowy hill, it becomes a large *muddied globe* at the bottom. So it is that our *magnetic minds* rapidly attract negative or positive thoughts, depending on the thought images or "*vibrations*" we project.

Vibrations are energy. They create a motive force, pulling together *more of the same,* positive or negative, like magnets pulling in the same direction. These negative or positive poles can be observed and applied in both tangible and intangible ways. We can optimize our health and prosperity almost effortlessly when we apply the L.O.A. Once we see how to effectively operate it, it becomes as effortless as sledding down a snow white hill. Like the wind accelerates the speed of a plane beyond its own ability, so we escalate by this amazing *tail wind* of the *L.O.A.* We soar in faith on the wings of *words* and *images.*

How do we give our attention, energy, and focus to attract what we desire, such as health and prosperity? Consider that the stars and sand continually before Abraham were tangible elements that supported his faith. The principles of the L.A.O. are ways to put what we see, feel, and hear into our immediate surroundings, to give more *attention* to what we desire. First, however, let's see how we *unintentionally* give attention to what we *don't want*, with words and observations.

When you say the word "travel," you might feel happy or stressed. What's important is how you *feel* about the words you speak and the images you see. Feelings create *vibrations*, or vibes as we say, which attract more of the same.

Therefore, when we change our words, we change our vibrations. By rewording negative phrases to a positive format, we change our vibration and, consequently, what we attract. There are three words that bring our attention to what we *don't want* — they are "don't," "not," and "no."

For example, if you say, "Don't think of rain," your mind unconsciously thinks of rain. Thus, when we rephrase it to say, "Think of a sunny day," we are shifting to a positive format. Here are common examples of how we can rephrase our daily conversations:

Common Phrases	**Rephrased**
Don't hesitate to call	Please call
Don't lose my number	Please keep my number
Don't be late	Please be on time
I'm not worried	I am confident
No rush	Take your time

When you hear yourself speak in the negative mode, simply ask yourself, "What do I want?" When you change your *words*, you change your *vibration*.

The words we speak and images we see generate emotions that create vibrations we send out. Words and images are encapsulated in our feelings, and feelings emit *vibrations*. The *vibration* that we send out comes back to us, causing us to have more of the same. We can only send out one vibration at a time, which reflects only how you feel at that moment.

Another way that we *unintentionally* give heed to what we *don't want* is in *observation*. We might observe a lack, such as viewing a low balance in our online savings account. As you observe, you are sending out a negative vibration. The L.O.A. responds to the *vibration* you are sending. Therefore, the key is *how long* we observe what we don't want.

For example, we might flip to a TV station that we quickly realize we don't want to see and click to the next. Yet, in other areas of our lives, we might observe or dwell on something far too long, such as a bad relationship or experience, thus inviting more of the same. It's important to observe the negative conditions as briefly as possible.

The L.O.A. responds to the vibrations you are sending by giving you more of the same, positive or negative. It simply responds to your current vibration. At every moment, you have a feeling or mood to which you emit a negative or positive vibration.

Identify the vibration you are sending and make a conscious choice whether you want to keep sending it or change it.

Your current vibrations are mirrored by the results you're getting in that area of your life. Your outcomes are a reflection of your vibrations. When you are complaining or talking about what you don't like, you're offering a negative vibration, but celebrating or discussing what you do like offers a positive vibe. The L.O.A. simply responds to give back more of the same. Let's now see how to raise our vibrations, which raises our faith, and receive our full bounty, as presented by Michael Losier in the *3 Steps for Deliberate Attraction*.

First - Identify Your Desire

Sounds easy, but it may actually be easier to know what you *don't want* than what you *do want*. Therefore, identify your desire by contrast. Contrast is anything you don't like, doesn't feel good, or causes you to be in a negative mood. Use contrast to become clearer about what you *do* want, as in the following Contrast/ Clarity worksheet:

Briefly observe contrast without getting stuck there. Often we observe contrast far too long in critical areas such as relationships, health, finance, and career. In these areas, many observe negative emotions, even for years.

Identify what makes you feel good and invite more of it. It's important to give yourself permission to feel good in all areas of your life. Choose an area of your life that you would like to improve or achieve.

Health, energy, strength

Career, clients, referrals

Income, savings, investments

Education, degree, certification

Friendships, marriage, self-esteem

Contrast/Clarity Worksheet

On the left side, list all of the things you don't like about your current or past experience of your ideal ____. Take time to make specific, brief descriptions. The more contrasts, the greater clarity. Select the heading as "Your desired ____ (health, career, soulmate, etc.)."

Contrast - list what you don't like **Clarity- list the things you would like**

Health:

Feeling fatigue	Feeling energy
Overweight	Moderate weight
Frequently sick	Usually well
Career:	
Bored with work	Fulfilled with work
Too many hours	Balanced hours
Long commute	Short commute
Soulmate:	
Non-expressive	Fully expressive
Selfish	Generous
Lives far away	Lives nearby

Cross out the left side as you convert each item to what you do want, which is the opposite, as in these examples. This will give you a clear focus of what you do want. The clearer your vision, the more likely you will acquire it.

Second - Give Your Desire Attention

Identify your desire and continue to give it attention. Giving attention to your desire increases *vibration*. Raise your vibration simply by giving more positive attention, energy, and focus, which brings you more of what you do want.

Imagine a vibration bubble surrounding you, capturing all your vibrations. Include your goals, dreams, and desires inside of your vibration bubble by putting them in arm's distance, or in some tangible way in front of you (like the sand and stars).

Vibration Bubble Worksheet

Create your Bubble worksheet to realize what raises your vibrations, with a list of what increases it on the left side, and decreases on the right side. Include what is in harmony with your desire on the left side, and the opposite on the right side. For instance, the left side might include pictures of a healthy, vibrant body, success reports, and affirmations. The right side would be a list of what brings negative attention, such as complaining, worrying, and doubting.

Raise Your Vibration

An affirmation is a statement spoken in present tense, declaring a desire, like "I have a balanced body." However, if that feels like an unattainable goal, or isn't true, saying it will give you a *negative vibration*. A positive affirmation can produce a negative vibration. The L.O.A. doesn't respond to words, but to how you *feel* about what you are saying. L.O.A. responds to your feelings (vibes), so the words need to be *true for you* to make you feel good.

The process of manifestation actually begins when you begin to give your desire any positive attention, such as talking or writing about it. So, you can be in the process of any aspiration, even if you've just begun. This sentence will make you feel good, and is believable, at any stage of the process. When it's true for you, it feels good. When it feels good, you are sending positive vibrations, which bring *more of the same*.

Desire Worksheet

Create your Desire Statement with the qualities from your clarity list. This allows you to talk about your desire in a way that it is true for you. The opening might begin, "I'm in the process of attaining my optimum health," which allows you to then develop it and talk about as it is truly in progress, thus enabling you to put it inside of your bubble.

The closing statement might be, "The science of the L.O.A. is unfolding and orchestrating all that needs to happen to bring my desire to me; and the Lord is upholding me in this transformation for His glory." This brings your desire into your

Vibration Bubble, making you feel good about your affirmations.

Step 3 – Allow it

Allowing is the absence of negative vibrations. Doubt is a negative vibration, which is often created by limiting beliefs. A negative vibration can dilute or cancel a positive vibration. Allowing is the *doubt removal process*, in essence, *allowing is enacting faith.*

"Now faith is the assurance of things hoped for, the conviction of things not seen" (Hebrews 11:1).

You know you're allowing when you hear yourself say statements such as, "Maybe I can have or do this," or, "Now this feels possible."

The game "Kerplunk" demonstrates this analogy. The marbles on top represent desires, the sticks symbolize doubts, and fallen marbles become manifestations. When the sticks are removed, marbles fall into manifestation. Your desire is manifested according to how much you *allow* it.

The source of most doubt is from our own self-limiting beliefs. These are the reoccurring thought patterns, usually after the word "because." For example you might say, "I'd like to start my own business, but can't *because* I am too old, too young, or too broke..." What are your limiting beliefs?

Create Allowing Statement

Allowing statements help you lessen or remove doubt from self-limiting beliefs. They will encourage you to believe that you will attract your desire. You can make allowing statements by answering the following questions:

Is anyone currently doing or having what I want to do or have?

If so, how many people are doing this today and previously?

Write believable statements in 3rd person, because making reference to yourself can create more doubt.

For example, to *allow* healing for a particular condition, you might respond as follows: "I have heard of some people who have recently been healed of ___. Previously, hundreds have been healed of ___. Anyone can be healed of___."

You will know you are *allowing* when you feel a sense of relief and when evidence is showing up in your life, *even partially*. For instance, if you see or feel any improvement in your health, or if you're hoping to meet your ideal soulmate, and you begin meeting (dating) those who are *closer* to your desire, c*elebrate.* Celebrate all evidence, which brings *attention* to your desire. Below are practical ways to help you *allow*, using health and healing examples.

10 Ways to help you Allow

1. Celebrate the *proof.* Note even partial evidence of progress, such as diminishing symptoms, slightly more energy, or feeling more optimistic.
2. Record your *proof* which lessens doubt (write notes, keep a diary, send texts and pictures, or make verbal recognitions).
3. Express appreciation to others and in prayer, which projects positive vibrations.
4. Define your lack as, "I'm in the process of … (recovering from Osteoporosis)."
5. Create a strong positive emotion by saying, "I've decided…" (A decision confirming your desire statement, such as, "I've decided to use both natural and conventional healing methods as appropriate for my condition.")
6. Open possibilities by saying, "Lots can happen… (especially when I consider that many others have been healed of this ailment.)"
7. Ask for information, and research to learn more about desires

and raise excitement, such as calling an agency or looking online for solutions, reading materials, or videos.

8. Make an attraction box, bulletin board, special shelf, or establish a tangible place to put anything that reflects your desire.
9. Create openings in your files, schedules, or environment, such as a file for healing modalities for your condition.
10. In prayer, relinquish the whole process to the Lord.

Attract Health and Prosperity

Abundance is a feeling, and feelings increase vibration. Therefore, deliberately include the feeling of abundance in your vibrational bubble by recording evidence of prosperity. Become aware of many different sources, and include the vibration of abundance as often as possible in your bubble. Celebrate when you've attracted abundance in *any form*.

Abundance is blessings, such as someone gives you something, buys your lunch, provides a referral, does you a favor, or gives you a tip, raise, or even a kind note. No matter how small it seems, giving it positive attention will raise your vibration to receive more of the same. Likewise, acknowledging any progress in your health, such as more energy, better skin texture, or becoming more muscular invites more improvements.

3 Ways to Increase the Vibration of Abundance

11. Record any evidence of abundance, prosperity, or improved health.
12. Accept gifts (whenever appropriate) - this turns up the dial of your receiving.
13. Post pictures of abundance, such as a gift certificate, a large check you received, or any steps toward good health or healing.

As you see, there are many simple, fun ways to increase your vibration through words and images that channel the undercurrent of our emotions. Begin using these strategies for your ideal health, or in any area, and you will absolutely attract what you *spotlight* in your life.

Conversely, the L.O.A. works just as effectively and powerfully in the negative. For instance, the media plays continuous coverage of a tragedy, and often, within a short time, there is more of the same type of tragedy. Of course, the media is just doing what it's supposed to do – broadcasting, but it is the audience who determines how long they will observe and how long they will give it their attention, energy, and focus.

The L.O.A. is a dynamic *Genesis Gem* providing gemstones that we can grasp to help sustain our faith even over a long span of time, as with Abraham.

We can use it to attract production and prosperity in our environment, as Jacob so wisely applied positive visual imagery, projecting his desire to produce premium sheep.

Begin to use the L.O.A. deliberately to bring health and well-being into your life. You can download these free worksheets on www.lawofattractionworksheets.com. Michael Losier's *Law of Attraction* book is a short but mighty sword, incorporating the practical application of the *Sword of the Spirit,* as supported by many scriptures below that reflect health and prosperity by words and images. The following verse amazingly weaves in all three elements of the L.O.A.:

"... *Give attention to my words; Incline your ear to my sayings. Do not let them depart from your eyes; Keep them in the midst of your heart; For they are life to those who find them, And health to all their flesh*" (Proverbs 4:20-22 NAS).

Attention by *inclining* your ear to His Word...

Focus by *keeping* them in front of your eyes and in your heart

Energy by *finding* them

"Death and life are in the power of the tongue, and those who love it will eat its fruits" (Proverbs 18:21 ESV).

"There is one whose rash words are like sword thrusts, but the tongue of the wise brings healing" (Proverbs 12:18 ESV).

"...The words I have spoken to you — they are full of the Spirit and life" (John 6:63).

"Gracious words are like a honeycomb, sweetness to the soul and health to the body" (Proverbs 16:24 ESV).

"See, I have engraved you on the palms of my hands; your walls are ever before me" (Isaiah 49:16 NIV).

"Let us fix our eyes on Jesus, the author and perfecter of our faith... " (Hebrews 12:2).

"Write them on the doorposts of your house and on your gates" (Deuteronomy 6:9 NLT).

The L.O.A. is that which is posted on the doorpost of your heart. In *Divine Healing Made Simple*, the author shares a profound dream that exemplifies just how one's focus can bring sickness or health. In his dream, there were some patients, who, when leaving the hospital, completely closed their account with the hospital. They were not allowed to make future appointments, discuss their disease, or even think about it after they were healed, except to occasionally testify about their healing. These patients never became sick again.

Other patients chose to keep their account open and could continue discussing their disease or injury as long as they wanted. They could make follow-up appointments, track the progression of sickness, and make payment arrangements. These people always became sick again.

The two mindsets show different views of how one gives attention, focus, and energy to sickness, while the other, to wellness. For instance, one may take possession of sickness, referring to it as "my diabetes," while the other leaves the package at the door – and refuses to *sign* for it!

One accepts their sickness as their own cross to bear, while the other acknowledges that Christ already bore the cross as our complete substitute, thereby focusing on his cross, not theirs. This is not to deny the existence of disease, but rather to deny its power over us, because greater is He who is in us than any disease.

These two approaches are more symbolic than literal. Obviously, if we have a condition that requires medical follow-up, we should, but then spiritually, we close the account of sickness, because Jesus paid it in full!

In closing, I'll share my own story of healing by "fixing my eyes on Jesus." One day, long bright red streaks appeared across my torso. The doctor studied the pattern and determined that I had shingles. Every time I passed by the mirror, I looked sadly at the red lashes. Then, I heard an inner voice saying, "Stop looking at the streaks, and start looking at me." Immediately, I went into prayer where hope flowed into another command, "Get a second opinion." So I did.

I went to a dermatologist's office, which was full of *third world* furniture. I was greeted by a Jamaican doc with long dreads. I wondered what *he* would say. He immediately diagnosed it as poison ivy and prescribed the appropriate medicine, which quickly cleared it up.

In the next chapter, we'll see the *Great Physician's second opinion*. May the principles of divine healing become *our first opinion*. No condition is permanent – only God's Word is everlasting, and the truth of the Word is greater than the seeming reality of disease.

Health Coach Recommendations:

Is that which you think, talk, or wonder about what you want more of in your life? If not, simply switch gears by asking yourself, "So what do you want?" You can ask this same question of someone whose complaining to you.

When using the words, "don't," "not," or "no," flip the switch to the positive mode.

Identify your desire clearly by using the Contrast/Clarity worksheet.

Give your desires attention by talking and thinking about them in the affirmations and visuals that raise your vibration.

Allow your desire to manifest by removing the sticks of doubt, usually your own self-limiting beliefs.

Bring evidence of abundance into your vibrational bubble.

Recommended Reading:

Law of Attraction by Michael Losier
Divine Healing Made Simple by Praying Medic

But I will restore you to health
and heal your wounds,
declares the LORD.
(Jeremiah 30.17)

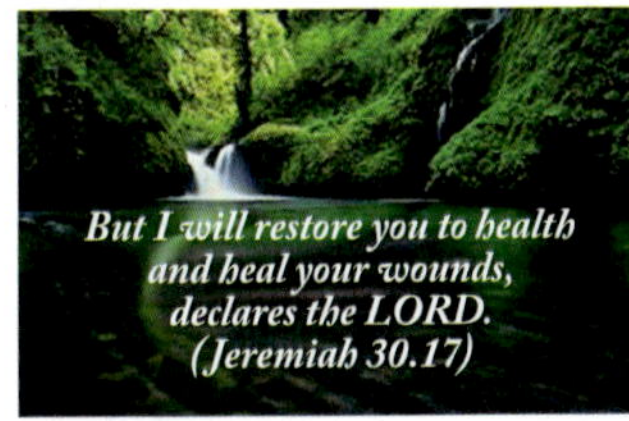

CHAPTER 11

The Law of Restoration

The principles of restoration are woven through the Genesis stories of Noah, Jacob, Joseph, Abraham and others. The L.O.A. is also intertwined throughout. The L.O.A. is also demonstrated in the lives of these patriarchs with *Perspective, Promise, Passion, Persistence, Patience, Positioning, Presence, and Performance.*

Perspective

When sick, we might ask, "Why are we suffering?" What is the physical cause? And at a deeper level, we might wonder, what is the spiritual cause? This is how Job's friends offered their *human insight.*

Consider now: Who, being innocent ever perished? Where were the upright ever destroyed? As I have observed, those who plow evil and those who sow trouble reap it" (Job 4:3-4). *Job's second friend continues, "As I have observed, those who plow evil and those who sow trouble reap it"* (Job 8:20 NIV). *Then his third friend reinforces the blame on Job, "If you put away the sin that is in your hand and allow no evil to dwell in your tent, then, free of fault, you will lift up your face; you will stand firm and without fear...Life will be brighter than noonday..."* (Job 11:14-15, 17).

One of the great barriers to receiving our healing is the human *blame game* — the same tactic purveyed by the *great accuser* in the Garden of Eden. Job's friends are much like our own internal dialogue, usually playing repeatedly until we shut it off by claiming God's promises. Like Job's friends who are focused on blaming rather than healing, so we witness this same tendency when Jesus was about to heal the blind man. However, Jesus penetrated through the clouds of human logic, presenting God's brilliant *aerial* point of view.

His disciples asked him, "Rabbi, who sinned, this man or his parents, that he was born blind?"

"Neither this man nor his parents sinned," said Jesus, "but this happened so that the works of God might be displayed in him" (John 9:2-4 NIV).

The Lord's perspective doesn't even grovel at the question of blame, but rather, shifts to the luminous glory of God. The following is my *blame* story, but soon shifted to *healing* glory.

My mother, 79, flew out to marry off yet another daughter – for that she never retires. After my wedding, my sister asked her to stay for a while. Two weeks later, as mother and I were walking out of the grocery store, I led her diagonally across the parking lot. As we crossed, she didn't see the speed bump, tripped, and tumbled onto the tarmac, severely breaking her hip. Over the next three months, mom's life took a traumatic turn.

It began with delayed hip replacement surgery, because it took a few days to adjust her blood thinning meds. After surgery, her hip popped out of place due to the rehab staff carelessly *man-handling* her. Thankfully, the surgeon was able to adjust it without too much discomfort.

Then she developed an infection when her body rejected the surgical staples. The infection grew rapidly worse. She felt her life slipping away. She cried out to God to save her. The next morning, her surgeon called to transfer her to an infectious disease specialist at Sinai Hospital in Baltimore. There, she finally began recovering.

My sister and I took turns staying with her, and during the long drive I would hear my "if onlys" play in my head. "If only I had led her straight, rather than diagonally, or if only I could have been more responsive and caught her… and if only we had not asked her to stay longer."

Then I started thinking about the blind man whom Jesus healed. When the disciples began asking, "Who sinned that this man was born blind?" Jesus put forth the most startling answer. It was not an answer to the *blame* question, where judgment resides in human logic, but rather an answer that comes from a far higher thought, above the cloud layer of humanity. "*This happened so the power of God could be seen in him*" (John 9:3). As I connected with this amazing truth, my "if onlys" were finally laid to rest.

Three months later, we took Mother to my sister's home as she continued in recovery. Two days after she arrived, however, she began to have extreme neck pain. There seemed to be no apparent cause, and when we took her back to the hospital, they still couldn't find any cause. The pain continually lingered. I knew then that often when there's no physical cause that can be found, the source is usually spiritual.

The next day, I went to see Mother. I was mad as hell at the devil! I asked her if I could pray for her. "Yes!" she said, most eagerly and grateful. I laid my hand on her neck and boldly spoke to the spirit of pain to leave immediately in Jesus name! I firmly spoke to it, just as I command my pit bull, and the *bully* left that very day!

Then I was able to assist Mother with another great leap of health. I took her to a natural hormone replacement specialist. Prior to this fall, Mother had also fallen a few times at home. Additionally, she had occasional debilitating back pain and resorted to steroid shots.

The doctor prepared customized natural hormone replacements and something wonderful began to happen. She became much better balanced, and her back began to straighten. Her appetite returned, and her frail body became strong again. Most amazing was the report of the bone density test, in less than two months after beginning therapy, showing a 50% improvement in her spinal bone mass!

I wept as I began to see over the cloud cover. Due to this trauma, she was made stronger than before. I stopped blaming, especially myself, and started praising; connecting with a higher thought that this happened so the power of God could be revealed in her life — Glory to God!

Beneath the layers of human blame of others (or our self) is unforgivenness. Throughout the scriptures, forgiveness is seen as a precursor to healing. Healing and forgiveness are presented as parallels, intricately connected.

"Praise the L*ORD, my soul, and forget not all his benefits, who forgives all your sins and heals all your diseases"* (Psalms 103-2, 3).

"He himself bore our sins in his body on the cross, so that we might die to sins and live for righteousness; by his wounds you have been healed" (1 Peter 2:24).

"Therefore confess your sins to each other and pray for each other so that you may be healed. The prayer of a righteous man is powerful and effective" (James 5:16).

"Which is easier: to say, 'Your sins are forgiven,' or to say, 'Get up and walk?'" (Luke 5:23).

We also experience healing as we share in Holy Communion, where Christ's blood was shed for the forgiveness of sin, and His body was broken for our healing. Our wholeness is equally the healing of our souls and of our bodies. Beyond the spiritual link of forgiveness and healing is a well-documented physical connection, as pastor Michael Barry unfolds.

In his book, *The Forgiveness Project: The Startling Discovery of How to Overcome Cancer, Find Health, and Achieve Peace*, Barry demonstrates the strong connection between the immune system and forgiveness. He shares stories of cancer patients experiencing spontaneous remission when they learn how to internalize forgiveness. According to the National Cancer Institute, *"chronic inflammation appears to contribute to tumor (growth) of different cancers."*

According to Barry, many may be unconscious of the unforgiveness we harbor. Sometimes we may carry this burden unaware of our own oppressed state, whether self-imposed or imposed on us by others. While we may be willing to forgive, we may not really know *how* to forgive. Forgiveness is not *ignoring* our pain, but rather, *releasing* our negative emotions to God. This is part of *The Forgiveness Project* whereby Barry helps the reader gain valuable insights.

In the Genesis story, they witness Joseph working through this process. Joseph, an amazing godly man, is also human. What begins as his brothers' manipulation seeking revenge for Joseph's favored status, ends in Joseph's understanding that all of his pain has been recycled for good, as he spoke from *The Lord's perspective*, *"You intended to harm me, but God intended it for good to accomplish what is now being done, the saving of many lives" (Genesis 50:20).*

Shifting now to another higher viewpoint is the *Promise*, that healing is for all people throughout all time.

Promise

How can we have faith for healing until we are absolutely sure that healing is still attainable for each of us today? We'll now explore the unwavering promises of Christ, who is the same yesterday, today, and forever. Notice the all-inclusive language wherever healing is mentioned; healing is for *everyone* from *every* disease or condition, in *every* age.

Beginning with the first covenant promise, after parting the Red Sea, as the conditions were fulfilled, "*He brought them forth also with silver and gold, and there was not one feeble person among their tribes" (Psalms 105:37).* From the beginning, the Lord established His relationship as Jehovah-Rapha, the healer.

Later, God provided healing for all by His word through Moses: *"So Moses made a bronze snake and put it up o a pole. Then when anyone was bitten by a snake and looked at the bronze snake, they lived"* (Numbers 21:9).

Then, the focus of Jesus' *entire ministry* was healing both the body and soul. Our compassionate Lord healed all who asked, even when He was exhausted, not turning *anyone* away.

As the sun went down that evening, people throughout the village brought sick family members to Jesus. No matter what their diseases were, the touch of his hand healed every one (Luke 4:40).

Jesus went through all the towns and villages, teaching in their synagogues, proclaiming the good news of the kingdom and healing every disease and sickness. When he saw the crowds, he had compassion on them… Jesus called his twelve disciples to him and gave them authority to drive out impure spirits and to heal every disease and sickness… Heal the sick, raise the dead, cleanse those who have leprosy, drive out demons. Freely you have received; freely give (Matt: 9:35, 36 and 10:1,8 NET).

The promise of healing extends to every person and includes every disease, every handicap, and every dysfunction. It includes shriveled extremities such as the man with the withered hand, mental illness, such as the epileptic boy; and birth defects, such as the man born blind. Furthermore, severed limbs growing back, is described in the healing ministry of Charles and Frances Hunter in their book, *"How to Heal The Sick"*, with explicit instructions in the chapter, "Growing out Arms and Legs" p. 157 -166. They explain how the restoration of a severed limb often cures other impairments that are connected to the damaged nerves, tendons, etc, such as severe back pain, deafness and blindness. When the limb grew out, they were also cured of the related ailment. On page 166, there are directions on how to heal yourself if even one limb is slightly shorter, such as a leg, which can alleviate back pain.

He even healed those whose loved ones made intercession for them, asking on their behalf, such as the centurion who asked for his servant, "…just say the Word and my servant will be healed."

The faith of the centurion did not require the physical presence of Christ, which would equate with our physical evidence of healing. He knew that the Lord's word alone imparts healing power.

Similarly, we implant the seed of the promise for our health and healing in our hearts by continually *watering* — speaking the promises that we are absolutely made whole. When we *pray* the promises, weaving the promises into our prayers, we are giving God's word back to Him, which never returns void. This becomes more dynamic and real as we personalize the promise in the present tense.

For instance, I used to have pain from a torn rotator cuff in my left shoulder. One day, I was doing gentle arm circles to rebuild my strength. I spontaneously said boldly out loud, "By your stripes I *was* healed, and I *am* healed, in Jesus name." At that moment the pain left, and I have had no further discomfort.

The following is a list of short healing promises that you can inscribe your name on and claim for your own, bringing them into reality.

"O Lord my God, I cried out to You, And You healed me" (Psalms 30:2).

"Bless the LORD, O my soul, And forget not all His benefits: Who forgives all your iniquities, Who heals all your diseases…" (Psalms 103:2).

"He sent His word and healed them, And delivered them from their destructions" (Psalms 107:20 NASB).

"He heals the brokenhearted And binds up their wounds" (Psalms 147:3).

"Do not be wise in your own eyes; Fear the Lord and depart from evil. It will be health to your flesh, And strength to your bones" (Proverbs 3:7, 8).

"But He was wounded for our transgressions, He was bruised for our iniquities; The chastisement for our peace was upon Him, And by His stripes we are healed" (Isaiah 53:5 KJV).

"Heal me, O LORD, and I shall be healed; Save me, and I shall be saved, For You are my praise" (Jeremiah 17:14 EST).

"For I will restore health to you And heal you of your wounds,' says the Lord..." (Jeremiah 30:17 AMP).

Is anyone among you sick? Let him call for the elders of the church, and let them pray over him, anointing him with oil in the name of the Lord. {15} And the prayer of faith will save the sick, and the Lord will raise him up. And if he has committed sins, he will be forgiven. {16} Confess your trespasses to one another, and pray for one another, that you may be healed. The effective, fervent prayer of a righteous man avails much (James 5:14-16).

What is the *prayer of faith?* It is the prayer that firmly upholds the promise of healing, as Jesus and the apostles demonstrated. This prayer believes that God not only has the ability to heal, but also is always *willing* to heal. When the leper asked if the Lord was willing, Jesus immediately confirmed His willingness, which remains the same today to anyone who asks.

"...Lord, if you are willing, You can make me clean." And He stretched out His hand and touched him, saying, "I am willing; be cleansed." And immediately the leprosy left him.... (Luke 5:12, 13).

Like the leper, it might be easy to believe that God has the power to heal, but still, one might feel unsure if He's willing to heal *you.* Personalizing God's promises makes them yours.

Knowing God's willingness greatly increases your expectancy. For instance, if you knew your name was included in your wealthy relative's inheritance, indicating their willingness to give to you, you would be convinced of receiving your inheritance. Their wealth (ability) may be impressive, but their willingness to pass it along to you builds your faith to receive. So it is with our spiritual inheritance. God zealously wants to give us wholeness of body and soul.

When you are convinced of God's strong desire to heal you, your language will change. Your prayers will not be preceded by the faith destroying words, *If you are willing, or if it be your will.* Look at the promises above. Is there any doubt that it is God's fervent desire that you are always completely healed?

The next piece of divine healing, *Passion,* will help you remove any sticks of doubt. This will help you *allow,* as discussed in the L.O.A. Once this doubt is removed, healing will begin to manifest in every area of life.

"Then your light will break forth like the dawn, and your healing will quickly appear..." (Isaiah 58:8). As you soak in these promises, the seed of God's word will sprout forth into health as promised, and faith will grow when you become, like Abraham, *fully persuaded* that healing is God's will for *you.*

<u>Passion</u>

We have seen that God is not only able, but is also willing to heal. Now we take this one step deeper. Not only is He willing, but He *passionately* wants to heal! Understanding His intense desire to heal raises your *vibration (as in the L. O.A.).*

When we hear the word passion associated with our Lord, we probably think of His Passion, i.e., the story of his final week and going to the cross to die for our sins. It is with this immense passion that Jesus laid down his life for his sheep. His passion was expressed as *compassion* during his earthly ministry that compelled him to heal everyone who asked. Now, as our High Priest, He continues with fervent desire to heal as the expression of God's will.

The LORD is merciful and compassionate, slow to get angry and filled with unfailing love (Psalm 145:8 NLT).

The words, compassion and mercy, have the same basic meaning in the scriptures and are used repeatedly to express God's passionate love. In the context of the great healing scriptures of James 5:14–16 is verse 11 portraying the heart of God for healing, as was seen for Job: "*...The Lord is full of compassion and mercy" (James 5:11).*

Throughout Jesus' ministry, we see how He was so filled with compassionate mercy that he continued to heal even when he was exhausted, even when he was taken captive by the soldiers, and even on His final moments on the cross, he spoke healing and forgiveness.

Our Lord poured out compassion on the overwhelming crowds, as He was equally merciful to each individual who came for healing. He never turned away anyone, and even when his disciples lacked the faith to heal, he continued until the man was made whole. Repeatedly, we see that Jesus healed *them all*, *everyone*, and *all who came to him*.

"He saw a great crowd and was moved with compassion toward them, and...He healed their sick (Matt. 14:14 BLT). … And when the men of that place had knowledge of him, they sent out into all that country round about, and brought unto him all that were diseased; And besought him that they might only touch the hem of his garment: and as many as touched were made perfectly whole" (Matt. 14:35, 36 KJV).

Since he was only one, and the multitudes multiplied, his tender mercies extended beyond himself, and he called the seventy to continue his healing ministry. As his disciples carried out his mission of love, many were spiritually saved after their physical healing. In fact, He promised that His work would be even greater after He went away, and that we shall do even greater works. It is the goodness of God that brings a man to repentance. The compassionate love of God inspires faith, healing both body and soul.

The Lord's compassion did not end with his earthly ministry, but he continues as our High Priest. He is moved by our sickness; still yearning to heal *all.* He is still touched by the feeling of our infirmities. Our High Priest still compassionately yearns to work through us, still touching the sick, and healing our infirmities.

"*Wherefore in all things it behooved him to be made like unto his brethren, that he might be a merciful and faithful high priest…*" (Hebrews 2:17 KJV).

For we have not a high priest which cannot be touched with the feeling of our infirmities; but was in all points tempted like as we are, yet without sin (Hebrews 4:15 KJV).

Imagine a mother compassionately sitting beside her sick child; she would do anything to help her child be well. Now imagine a love that far surpasses the extent of human compassion. That is our High Priest, *moved* by our illness and grief, which *moves* us to a higher plateau of faith.

This is our compassionate God who has engraved our names upon the palms of His hand, who knows the number of hairs on our head, and who sent His only son to endure what we could not. His love extends even to sinners; how much more to those who love Him?

"But the mercy of the LORD is from everlasting to everlasting upon them that fear Him, And His righteousness unto children's children…" (Psalm 103:17 KJV).

God's mercy is so great that he uses an incomprehensible measurement of time "from *everlasting to everlasting*" to tell of His incomprehensible love for us. He further expresses it by an inconceivable span of the universe, from *the east to the west*, taking our imagination for a spin "*…as far as the east is from the west, so far has he removed our transgressions from us*" (Psalm 103:12 KJV). What a metaphor of God's eternal love and forgiveness!

"For thou, Lord, art *good, and ready to forgive; and plenteous in mercy unto all them that call upon thee" (Psalm 86:5 KJV).*

In many cases, divine intervention occurs when we *call upon* or *cry out* for the Lord, as we *move* from complacency and tolerance to determination. This is when the Lord is *moved* by *our passion* for healing, just as when our children cry out to us in times of need.

I witnessed this powerful intercession when my mother was recovering from her hip replacement surgery. She felt her life slipping away as the infection spread. She was caught in a holding place because her surgeon was too far away, and the attending hospital physician was reluctant to engage in the midst of this issue. Mother cried out to the Lord in the middle of the night, and by the early morning, she was on the way to an infectious disease specialist where she began recovery.

Our God "delighteth in mercy" (Micah 7:18 KJV). As we comprehend His immense, intense love for us, how unfounded becomes the question, "if it be thy will." As we move to *Persistence,* the Lord returns the question back to us, asking, <u>"If it be *our* will?"</u>

<u>Persistence</u>

"Then Jacob was left alone; and a Man wrestled with him until the breaking of day. Now when He saw that He did not prevail against him, He touched the socket of his hip; and the socket of Jacob's hip was out of joint as He wrestled with him.

And He said 'Let me go be for the day breaks.' But he said, 'I will not let You go unless You bless me!' So He said to him, 'What is your name?' He said, 'Jacob.' And He said, 'Your name shall no longer be called Jacob, but Israel; for you have struggled with God and with men, and have prevailed.'

"So Jacob was left alone, and a man wrestled with him till daybreak. When the man saw that he could not overpower him, he touched the socket of Jacob's hip so that his hip was wrenched as he wrestled with the man. Then the man said, 'Let me go, for it is daybreak.' But Jacob replied, 'I will not let you go unless you bless me.' The man asked him, 'What is your name? Jacob,' he answered. Then the man said, 'Your name will no longer be Jacob, but Israel, because you have struggled with God and with humans and have overcome.' Jacob said, 'Please tell me your name.' But he replied, 'Why do you ask my name?" Then he blessed him there. So Jacob called the place Peniel, saying, 'It is because I saw God face to face, and yet my life was spared'" (Genesis 32:24-30 NIV).

Jacob did not mince words saying, "Bless me *if it be your will,*" but rather, he wrestles with the man (the angel) all night long. Still clenching the angel before daybreak, he insists, *"I will not let You go unless You bless me!"* Then he blessed him and changed his name to *Israel*, a name that signified his perseverance. Indeed, Jacob was a man of unwavering diligence; a man who served a double term for his prized bride and produced premium sheep from the runts of Laban's flock.

Persistence makes God smile. It produces the *works* spoken of in James 5: "without works faith is dead." It promotes the *greater works* that Jesus prophesied, *"... Whoever believes in me will do the works I have been doing, and they will do even greater things than these, because I am going to the Father"* (John 14:12).

Persistence doesn't give up, give in, or give out, but rather, it is a bull fighter (like Jacob) that holds onto its blessing no matter how many times it gets bucked off. It stretches our prayer, our perspective, and our endurance to grasp tight of the blessing already promised: our complete healing.

Jesus teaches us about persistence in two amazing parables, the parable of the persistent widow and the man asking for bread in the late night.

"Then Jesus told his disciples a parable to show them that they should always pray and not give up. He said, 'In a certain town there was a judge who neither feared God nor cared what people thought. And there was a widow in that town who kept coming to him with the plea, 'Grant me justice against my adversary."

"For some time he refused. But finally he said to himself, 'Even though I don't fear God or care what people think, yet because this widow keeps bothering me, I will see that she gets justice, so that she won't eventually come and attack me!'"

And the Lord said, *"Listen to what the unjust judge says. And will not God bring about justice for his chosen ones, who cry out to him day and night? Will he keep putting them off? I tell you, he will see that they get justice, and quickly. However, when the Son of Man comes, will he find faith on the earth?"* (Luke 18:1-8).

Since this woman is a widow, she has no husband to stand as her advocate and must therefore dig in her heels and fight for her rights or promise for justice. All the odds are against her because she is asking for *justice* from an *unjust* judge. She is so bold that she even scares the judge. (Got to love that lady!)

On the contrary, Jesus asks, wouldn't our *just* God (full of mercy and compassion) bring justice to his own who are *persistent*? He affirms that they will get justice (the blessings they are promised, such as healing). He then asks a question to ponder, "When the Son of Man comes, will he find faith?" This question is the sum of the whole parable: Will he find *this kind of persistent faith* that holds its own, standing as its own advocate in the face of adversity? Will He see this kind of faith for healing, even in the midst of the roaring lion of disease?

In the next parable, Jesus expounds the meaning further at the end of the story.

"He said to them, 'Which of you, if you go to a friend at midnight, and tell him, 'Friend, lend me three loaves of bread, for a friend of mine has come to me from a journey, and I have nothing to set before him,' and he from within will answer and say, 'Don't bother me. The door is now shut, and my children are with me in bed. I can't get up and give it to you?' I tell you, although he will not rise and give it to him because he is his friend, yet because of his persistence, he will get up and give him as many as he needs" (Luke 11:5-8 WEB).

"I tell you, keep asking, and it will be given you. Keep seeking, and you will find. Keep knocking, and it will be opened to you. For everyone who asks receives. He who seeks finds. To him who knocks it will be opened" (Luke 11:9-10 WEB).

In the first parable, the widow was persisting against an unjust judge, but here, Jesus says if you had such a friend who was unwilling to help in time of need, persistence would prevail.

There are few clues in this short analogy where Jesus teaches the fullness of persistent faith. First the man comes at midnight. God tells us to come boldly to the throne of grace in prayer any time, for anything according to his will. Also, God calls us His *friend*, but He does not answer our prayer on the basis of our friendship, but because of His covenant with us. Relationships can teeter, but God's relationship with us is unchanging.

Then Jesus clearly describes persistence, which is standing at the door *until you receive*. He states the promise, "*Search and you will find; knock and the door will be opened for you*" (Luke 11:9-10 WEB). He is not referring to the pesky salesman persistence that can't take "no" for an answer, but rather the ability to stand firmly on the promises of God that always takes "Yes" as *the answer*, before the door even opens. "Yes," I have already received healing, even if I don't see it yet. It continues to say, "*Yes,*" until healing manifests, no matter what the *current conditions* appear to be.

There are two more great stories of healing by persistent *knocking*, but not knocking at the door. The first is about a paralyzed man who cannot get through the crowds to be brought to Jesus. He convinces the men carrying him to lower him by *knocking* a hole through the ceiling!

And they brought to Him a paralytic lying on a bed. Seeing their faith, Jesus said to the paralytic, "*Take courage, son; your sins are forgiven … Get up, pick up your bed and go home.*" And he got up and went home (Matt. 9:2 -7 NASB).

Not only did the man demonstrate audacious faith by coming *through the ceiling*, but when he took the action of getting up, he was healed. That is the same way we demonstrate faith for our healing. This man's body was *paralyzed*, but in no way was his faith.

The second story is about a woman who had a bleeding disorder for 12 years. Can you imagine how weak she must have felt? Yet this woman was adamantly *knocking*, too. In fact, she was probably *knocking* people over to get to Jesus. Her faith was so determined that she didn't even need to physically touch Jesus, just his garment. She knew that His power was real and was for her!

Knock and keep on knocking. If there is no answer, climb through the window, slither though the cellar, or descend through the attic. The door will open as you speak the promises of healing and take the corresponding action.

Stand firm on your confession, no matter how turbulent the waves are tossing about. There will always be waves, but when you persistently ride with the waves, giving thanks and praise to God who is the great calmer of the seas, the waves will no longer trouble you.

"But let him ask in faith, without wavering, for he who wavers is like the waves of the sea which the wind troubles…" (James 1:6 ABPE).

Persistent faith is like a surfer, standing firmly and soaring on *top* of the water, and though falling *seven times*, it gets back up, and keeps on keeping on, believing God for what He has already promised.

What kinds of faith will the Son of Man find when He returns?

Patience

Patience is yoked to persistence; these two powerful stallions run together, upholding faith.

God promises that when we pray, "They shall recover," but not necessarily *immediately*. It may occur immediately, miraculously, or it may materialize some time afterwards. The point of healing is not *when we see it*, but *when we pray*. We believe that we *have received when we pray* with words and actions corresponding to our prayer.

Therefore I tell you, whatever you ask for in prayer, believe that you have received it, and it will be yours (Mark 11:24).

We are to believe that we *have* received. When Jesus came to Lazarus, even days after he died, he said, "I thank thee, Father, that thou *hast* heard me." Jesus is our model for appropriating healing, and raising the dead is certainly the ultimate demonstration of God's restorative power. Though symptoms and pain may linger, we know we are already restored. We continue to speak it into being, "I am *in the process of* complete recovery." Divine healing happens "when we pray," regardless of what we see or feel. Patience is the horse that wins the race.

But if we hope for what we do not yet see, we wait for it patiently (Romans 8:25).

If a judge granted you a large sum of money in a courtroom, you legally received the benefit *the moment he spoke the order*, although it may be months or even years before you actually have it. How much more can we be assured that what God has *ordered* in the heavenly courts will come to pass? And here is where we turn to our *great cloud of witnesses.*

The promised seed took many years to be fulfilled through Abraham and Sarah, whereas with Mary, the mother of Jesus, it happened instantly. The Lord challenges us to trust Him to perform a miracle in our physical bodies, whether the seeds of healing sprout immediately or over time.

"And so after waiting patiently, Abraham received what was promised" (Hebrews 6:15).

Likewise, Noah's patience stretched during an unfathomable 120 years of persecution while building what looked like a useless vessel; then he waited for more than another whole year *in* the ark. Job, too, endured such excruciating pain and losses; still he chose to honor and wait upon the Lord. He was not only healed but received a double blessing.

"For ye have need of patience, that, after ye have done the will of God, ye might receive the promise" (Hebrews 10:36 KJV).

Patience is like piers sunk deeply into bedrock that supports our faith. The longer our bridge, the more piers we need. The higher the structure, the more deeply and firmly it must be grounded. Prayer, scriptures, and reflections of His marvelous works are our greatest *piers*. Reflecting on what He has done helps us trust in what He will do.

Healing scriptures are the seed that we implant in our hearts, that will absolutely mature so long as we keep it planted and not *dig it up* with doubt. We dig up the seed when we worry, complain, and give more attention to symptoms than to the healing promises. Know that He who created the seed gave it the ability to germinate, grow, and produce what was intended from the beginning — the fruitful harvest of God's goodness that is meant for all. God assures us of a harvest, so long as we don't give up.

"But that on the good ground are they that, in an honest and good heart, having heard the Word, keep it and bring forth fruit with patience" (Luke 8:15 KJV).

"Let us not become weary in doing good, for <u>at the proper time</u> we will reap a harvest if we do not give up" (Gal.6:9).

<u>Positioning</u>

In *Christ the Healer*, F.F. Bosworth explains that divine healing (and any blessing) is like *positioning* yourself in a game of checkers. Players must wait their turn until the others play.

God has made the first move by providing healing through His word. Our move is to expect what He has promised, *by looking at Christ when* we pray. The Israelites were instructed to *look* upon the brazen serpent (a type of a*tonement* for bodily healing) just as God's Word (as fully expressed by Jesus) is our a*tonement* for bodily healing. In this sense, *look* means to be fully occupied, giving full attention, with expectation and careful consideration.

It is the continuous present tense. Then, the next move is God's — His healing. He never moves out of turn, but always moves when it is His turn. We position ourselves to receive.

Another way we position ourselves for healing is to remove hindrances. When a strong batter comes up to home plate, the outfielder moves back, away from anything blocking reception, positioning himself to catch a long fly ball. So we position ourselves, moving ourselves from the obstacles that might prevent us from *catching* God's healing grace. The following are some reasons that some fail to receive healing, as presented by F.F. Bosworth in his book, *Christ the Healer*(paraphrased).

Insufficient instruction can prevent healing because we must be fully persuaded that healing for everyone is God's absolute will, just as much as it is for salvation. "*...Faith comes by hearing, and hearing by the word of God*" (Romans 10:17 AKJV). Nothing builds one's faith as much as when they hear *their self* say, and read, God's healing promises. If you are in need of healing (as truly we all are in some way), this is where we must begin. It can only grow in the *good ground* when we learn it, allow it to *penetrate* into our spirit, and *keep* this *imperishable* seed planted until we see it manifest.

The traditions of men can void God's healing power. Jesus told the authorities that they were *"making the word of God of no effect through your tradition"* (Mark 7:13 KJ2000B). Not much has changed today. These traditions have become stumbling blocks to receive healing, such as the belief that "the age of miracles has passed." How could that be when Jesus said this would be the time of *greater works?* Another misconstrued belief is that we "glorify God by our affliction." Yet, Jesus always glorified the Father by healing, not by sickness, as He affirmed many times. The other myth is that it is not God's will to heal all or all diseases. How can this be when healing every one and every disease clearly echoes throughout the entire Bible?

Unforgiveness is another barrier. As unforgiveness is bound to healing, so is our *need to seek forgiveness.* Our own forgiveness is contingent upon forgiving others. Jesus made this clear by saying it in both the positive and the negative form, the reward or consequence. *And without faith it is impossible to please Him, for he who comes to God must believe that He is and that He is a rewarder of those who seek Him."* (Matt 6:14-15 NASB). He further drives home this principle with the emotionally charged story of the unforgiving servant. Perhaps one of the links between healing and forgiveness is that when we forgive, or seek forgiveness of others, we experience the full manifestation of God's forgiveness to us. Many have been miraculously healed as soon as they were released from the spirit of unforgiveness.

Lack of Diligence or Desire prevents many from being healed. God rewards those who seek healing diligently and wholeheartedly. Unfortunately, some have alternative motives such as remaining in their pity, lack of self-love, or receiving financial compensation. There is never a question of God's diligence or desire. That question is only for the recipient. Jesus often gave commands to those he healed whereby they demonstrated their diligence by obedient faith, such as to get up, go wash in the pool, or put mud on their eyes.

"But without faith, it is impossible to please Him, for he who comes to God must believe that He is, and that He is a rewarder of those who diligently seek Him" (Hebrews 11:6 NKJV).

By breaking the natural *laws of health,* we are violating the divine principles of nature. When we harmonize with them, it's easy to trust for preventive health and restoration. If, however, we are regularly consuming toxins from excess sugar, it will be difficult to expect health. God established himself as *our physician* and *our health coach* with dietary and health recommendations throughout His word, like the many we reviewed earlier.

Sometimes, *spiritual influence must be removed* when an affliction is the attack of an evil spirit. Jesus cast out the epileptic spirit and deaf, dumb, and blind spirits. Often when there can be no medical reason for an issue, the cause is demonic. Jesus says "in my name they shall cast out demons." Many have been instantly healed when the afflicting spirit was rebuked.

As Peter's faith was weakened when he looked down at the waves, so is ours as we *look down at our symptoms*. God's Word is our basis for healing, not what we see or feel. When we keep our eyes steadfast on the promise, as did Abraham, the impossible becomes reality. When we wait for healing before we believe, we have reversed the conditions. Rather, once we pray, we rejoice with thanksgiving that we *have been healed*. If we truly believe, we will pray for our healing *only once,* and then our prayers are of worship and thanksgiving, knowing we have already received.

Fortunately, we are not doomed by our own unbelief, but we can cry out to the Holy Spirit to help us overcome our unbelief. Immediately the boy's father exclaimed, "I do believe; help me overcome my unbelief!" (Mark 9:24). Furthermore, speaking faith affirmations such as, "You will be healed in Jesus Name," builds confidence.

Finally, inviting the Holy Spirit to fill us with His fullness positions us for healing. Although we all received the Holy Spirit at our new birth, we still invite the Holy Spirit into our *living temple*. As we invite Him into our heart, our home, our workplace, and everywhere we go, we bring with us His healing presence. In prayer, or at any moment, we can ask the Holy Spirit for a *refill, which* allows His healing power to cascade from *our* presence.

Presence

When we remove these obstacles, we will walk on healing waters. Since the Holy Spirit is the healer, we invite His presence when we pray for healing. His presence within a faith-filled believer empowers restoration, as in the early church.

The church in the book of Acts is our blueprint from when it had an outpouring of the Holy Spirit throughout the whole church. *"All these continued together in prayer with one mind…"* (Acts 1:14 NET). This produced such a Spirit-filled atmosphere that many were healed, for example, just from the shadow of Peter passing by. The power was in the Spirit-filled atmosphere, the essence of the Holy Spirit that was imparted by Peter's shadow and Paul's handkerchief. Christians are commanded to pray together for the outpouring of the Holy Spirit, which causes us to prevail in prayer for the sick. The *community's faith* causes the tide to rise or fall for inviting God's power in healing. Even Christ, fully anointed by the Holy Spirit, could not do many mighty works in his hometown because of their unbelief.

Performance

Then the LORD said to me, "You have seen well, for I am watching over my word to perform it" (Jeremiah 1:12 ESV).

God said He is watching over His word to perform it. It was not Jeremiah, but God who would perform it. When asking for divine healing, this is the childlike confidence that God honors, knowing that He is eager to perform His word in us. He yearns for our healing even more than we do, and nothing glorifies Him more. It is His power flowing through our hands, His Spirit is behind our words, His compassion spilling over from our hearts, and His energy rejuvenating our mortal bodies.

The Holy Spirit is the healer who always heals, but we open the pathways in the many ways we have discussed in this chapter. We shift from our human *perspective* of shame to the godly viewpoint of glorifying God. As we forgive and receive forgiveness, we open the gateway to healing. Forgiveness is the beginning of God's *passionate* love for us. He poured out His life because He is just as *compassionate* about healing our bodies as our souls. He fills us with His healing *presence* at any time we ask. When we are *fully persuaded* of His promises, we no longer lose confidence by adding, "If it be thy will," for we know that it is God's will to keep his promises.

Real faith is *persistently patient.* It is like a fox that tirelessly waits for its game to come out of the hole. Though he cannot see the little animal inside its den, he stands sure that it is inside and will surface eventually. Therefore, he doesn't give up or give in, but will take what he's sure is already his. So our persistent faith knows that the doors of blessings and healing will open when we knock. That which we ask (according to His will), we will receive, and that which we seek, we will find, "exceedingly abundantly above all that we could ask or think."

Finally, we *position* ourselves on wings of the Lord; and He renews our strength like the eagles. We remove the weights that prevent us from soaring in His healing power, such as the myths of men, unforgiveness, and focusing on symptoms. Like Jonah, while still in the whale's belly, we offer the sacrifice of thanksgiving. What greater demonstration of faith than when we are giving thanks before we see or feel our healing?

Health Coach Recommendation:

Restoration through Forgiveness

In *The Forgiveness Project,* author and Pastor, Michael Barry, shares profound insights that have helped many achieve peace, health, and even overcome cancer. Yet, understanding what is forgiveness, and how to process it, may be obscure, even for many Christians.

Barry first addresses some misunderstandings about what forgiveness is, and is not. First, what it is NOT:

It is not mental consent, or lip service, but rather, a change of heart whereby we release resentment, anger, and hatred to the Lord, which He replaces with His perfect peace.

It is also not forgoing justice, meaning that the offender should still be accountable for their actions, but we place the staff of justice in God's hand, not ours.

It does not necessarily imply reconciliation. In fact, you need never to speak to them again. If someone is dangerous or toxic, no further interactions may be best.

Forgiveness is an emotional shift. It's like putting all the negative emotions in the basket of a hot air balloon, and in prayer, cutting each rope that anchors it to your heart. These ropes may be emotional and or physical abuse, resentment, or anger. Once released, a feeling of lightness, a cheerful heart is now released, like the balloon into the sky.

Barry suggests that one of the best ways to begin this process is to write a letter to your adversary, explaining how they hurt you, and the implications of their actions or words. Write in detail to express as fully as you can, but do not give it to them. It is only for you, as a means of releasing these toxic emotions. Barry shares that many have been healed of cancer and other disease after releasing this *emotional inflammation.* The typical cancer patient, Barry says, has a type "C" personality. "C" stands for Chronic niceness, and Conflict avoidance. They consequently suppress feelings to avoid conflict. This inflammation eventually manifests in the physical.

Jesus was, and still is our amazing example of forgiveness. In His healing ministry, He not only forgave, but also restored each one he forgave, both physically and spiritually. At the last supper, He forgave his offenders before they even carried out their unthinkable wrongdoings.

In the midst of His own anguish, He forgave one of the Roman soldiers by healing his ear, an incredible act of forgiveness! While hanging in excruciating pain on the cross, He forgave those beside Him. And in His final words, He forgave those "who know not what they do". Who of us really knows the extent, and ripple effect of *"what we do"?*

Barry further explains that we tend to dehumanize our offenders, thereby, making ourselves better, a subtle form of self-righteousness. We like to lick our wounds and tell others about our awful offender. Yet, to truly forgive, we must see their *humanity.* Though we may never do something as evil, or wrong as they did, we too have hurt others. In our humility, we see their humanity. When we see their humanity, we can begin to feel empathy for our offender. *Empathy* then leads to understanding and forgiveness. Indeed, forgiveness is a project!

The measure of forgiveness, Barry says, is if you feel that you could sincerely wish them well. Jesus tells us to pray for our enemies. When we do, ironically, we release not them, but *ourselves*, our pains, our chains, and possibly freeing us from the power of disease.

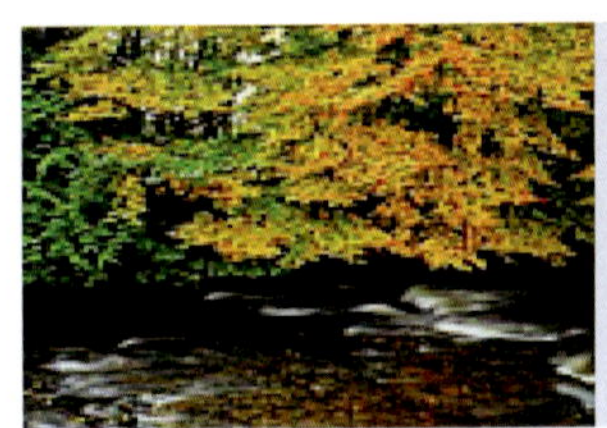

Chapter 12
The Law of Fulfillment

"They are like trees planted along the riverbank, bearing fruit each season. Their leaves never wither, and they prosper in all they do" (Psalm 1:3 NLT).

Genesis closes the curtains with Joseph, a man whom the Lord escalated from behind the bars — to shine as the stars, once a cell mate, then, the head of Pharaoh's estate!

Here, the last two gems of Genesis are illuminated, not in the earth or sky, but in the heart and soul: values and dreams, as portrayed in Joseph's life of many colors. We'll see how Joseph's values and dreams carried him to his purpose and destiny, and likewise for us.

Joseph lived by his values of integrity, spirituality, reverence and resourcefulness, as seen in his dealings with Potiphar's wife, Pharaoh, his cellmates, and in his leadership. He was fulfilled in every way in spite of the harsh circumstances:... *"For God has made me fruitful in the land of my affliction."* (Genesis 41:52 ESV)

We too can be fulfilled as we discover our values, and understand our dreams. Beyond the surface level of happiness, with aspirations of wealth, health, and a fitting career or lifestyle, is the center of our hearts. There, our *values* bring us *full joy*. As we live out our values, we become *fully alive*! These qualities awaken our soul, because they are our soul life!

When we live in harmony with our values, we live genuinely — with integrity by who we are, not what we're *supposed* to be or think we *should* be. Instead, we start living from the inside out, in our full potential. When you unveil your values, you become the real you; synchronized with your life's purpose. Michael

Losier's "Fulfillment Needs" training program, along with other methods that I will share, can help you discover yours. I consider *fulfillment needs* and *values* essentially the same and use them interchangeably.

Values are what you believe is important in your life. They are the measuring stick of our joy. We feel deep joy when what we do and think reflects our values in our work, career, leisure, or lifestyle, but when we're out of alignment with our personal values, we simply don't thrive. For instance, if one of your core values is integrity, but you work for a company that is not upfront with their customers, you feel continual tension and compromise.

As we realize our values, it's easier to determine our priorities, and live in our life's purpose. They guide us in answering important questions as to which is the best choice when considering what type of career, or if starting a new business, accepting a promotion, or doing volunteer work. As our definition of success changes, so do our values. Therefore, keeping in touch with our current fulfillment needs helps us to be balanced and fulfilled.

If you feel that your life is unfulfilling, unearth your values. If you're not sure what your values are, you can scan the lists of values online or below and circle the qualities that bring strong emotions or propel you toward action.

Accomplishment
Accuracy
Achievement
Adventurousness
Art
Assertiveness
Balance
Boldness
Cleanliness
Challenge
Cheerfulness
Commitment
Community
Compassion
Competitiveness
Consistency
Contentment
Contribution
Control
Cooperation
Correctness
Courtesy
Creativity
Curiosity
Decisiveness
Dependability
Determination
Devoutness
Diligence
Discipline
Diversity
Economy
Effectiveness
Efficiency
Elegance
Empathy
Enjoyment
Enthusiasm
Equality
Excellence
Expertise
Exploration
Expressiveness
Fairness
Faith
Family
Fidelity
Fitness
Freedom
Fun
Generosity
Goodness
Growth
Happiness
Hard Work
Health
Honesty
Honor
Humility
Independence
Ingenuity
Inquisitiveness
Insightfulness
Intelligence
Intuition
Joy
Justice
Leadership
Legacy
Love
Loyalty
Mastery
Merit
Obedience
Openness
Order
Originality
Patriotism
Perfection
Positivity
Practicality
Preparedness
Professionalism
Prudence
Quality
Reliability
Resourcefulness
Security
Self-control
Sensitivity
Serenity
Service
Simplicity
Spirituality
Spontaneity
Stability
Strategic
Strength
Structure
Success
Support
Teamwork
Temperance
Thankfulness
Thoroughness
Thoughtfulness
Timeliness
Tolerance
Traditionalism
Trustworthiness
Truth-seeking
Understanding
Uniqueness
Unity
Usefulness
Vision
Vitality

Narrow it down to eight: four primary and four secondary. If you see that some are very closely related, they could be tagged together as one. The following questions can help define your bullseye values.

1. When did you feel the most joyful? What were you doing, who were you with, and what was the environment?
2. When did you feel the most honored? What were you doing, who were you with, and what was the environment?
3. When did you feel the most content? What were you doing, who were you with, and what was the environment?

Which values are reflected in each experience? This will help you whittle down to the more important ones. The next three questions will help you to further identify the top four fulfillment needs.

1. What are four things that you don't like about your current job, and what are four things you do like about it?
2. What are four things that you don't like about your volunteer work, and what are four things you do like about it?
3. What are four things that you didn't like about your past relationship, and what are four things you do like about your current relationship?

Look for reoccurring qualities that you like and dislike which point to your fulfillment needs or values. They should be priorities in your life and what you give the most *attention*, *focus*, and *energy* to because they will bring you the greatest joy. Conversely, you won't waste precious time and energy on what is not in sync with your values.

As we are learning, the Law of Fulfillment (L.O.F.) reveals what you really want, your *soul needs*. Here is how I used these wonderful tools to achieve health and happiness in two major areas: meeting my soul mate, and developing a writing career.

First, I recognized that my primary values were *creativity, accomplishment, health, and spirituality*; and my secondary values were *organization, cleanliness, community, and compassion.* Together, they are like the pilot (primary) and co-pilot (secondary) soaring in balance.

I was 49 when I finally met my soul mate. By then, I had lots of experience to know what I *didn't* want, which helped me become clear about what I *did* want.

I stopped *window shopping* and started to look *within*, at my personal values. Then it all became clear that the best guy for me is the one who is in *harmony* with my values. Indeed, his fulfillment needs mirrored and beautifully complemented mine.

I prayed, submitting the whole matter to the Lord, with a profile that captured some of my values and reflected my personality in a creative prose form. By giving my *attention, focus,* and *energy* to what I am, I naturally attracted the same qualities in my partner.

When we live by our own values, we bring our whole selves into the relationship. I believe that relationships are the core of our well-being. They can boost our immune system or drain it. They can elongate our lifespan or shorten it. Whatever we give our attention, focus, and energy to within our marriage, we reap more of the same.

Also, I was guided by my values in my aspiration for writing, which helped me break through my self-limiting beliefs. I used *reasoning* regarding my current success to remove the *sticks of doubt.* I reminded myself that "Since I am good with creative solutions in my business, I can just as easily be a *creative* writer. Since I have the organizational skills and persistence to stay in business, I can finish a book!" My values of health, compassion, and spirituality also moved me through an occasional writer's block. It was then that I felt a steady stream of thoughts and words flowing from a limitless reservoir.

Likewise, dreams spring forth our fulfillment, as seen in Joseph's life. God portrayed Joseph's great destiny to him, even when he was young, many years prior to their manifestation.

Then Joseph told his brothers. *'Listen,' he said, 'I had another dream, and this time the sun and moon and eleven stars were bowing down to me.'* (Genesis 37:9 NLT)

At this time, Joseph didn't understand the vision that was embedded in his heart, which would take a lifetime to unfold. This is the secret language of the Lord to the dreamer. Joseph's father misinterpreted the symbolism of the sun and moon to be his parents, but God was giving Joseph His global vision!

Similarly, the Lord prepares us for our divine purpose and fulfillment through dreams, visions, and imagery. Since both the dream and interpretation come from God, we need to learn God's picturesque language, through His Word, to decode His thoughts. More than one third of the Bible is symbolism and metaphorical language, such as proverbs, prophesy and parables. Words easily slip away, but images become engraved in our soul, imparting the full emotional impact — that ripples deeply into our heart, in night parables.

Dream interpretation is similar to literary interpretation, and is guided by the Holy Spirit. Therefore, the Spirit of the Lord is the pilot, and logic is the co-pilot. As we develop metaphorical thinking and a journalistic mind, we cultivate accurate dream interpretation. Ultimately, the Lord provides the meaning.

By journalistic mind, I'm referring to the five W's questions of a journalist: who, what, when, where, and why. These answers provide context, and to whom and what area of life it applies. As accurate interpretation encompasses the whole picture surrounding literary excerpts, so it is in dreams. The context of the dream points to a specific area of our lives; and the context of our lives, directs us to the application. Spiritual dream interpreter, Doug Addison coaches by asking these important four questions:

First, who or what is the dream about, and what area of your life does it pertain to? If you are in the dream, is the spotlight on you, or are you just involved, participating, or observing? If you are on center stage, it's likely about you; or if about you and someone or something else, it may be about you and them or it. If you're observing, it's more likely about what you're observing. Observing dreams often reveal someone we should support and pray for. What area of your life does it point to? Are the characters in your dream, your family or church members, or associated with your work, school, or recreation? The setting is a clue as to what part of your life the dream is highlighting, where, or with whom it occurs, and when — present, past or furture.

Second, how is the dream visualized? Are the colors bright or dark, muted or clear? This sets the tone — positive or negative. In bright dreams, God is often encouraging or birthing something new, and in some dark dreams, He may be showing us areas of our life that need change. Dull or muted color dreams, may be about plans of darkness against you, or your own fears. Dark dreams and nightmares can be "flipped around" to a positive application, as Addison shares in his book, *Understanding Your Dreams Now: Spiritual Dream Interpretation.*

Third, is it a reoccurring dream, or a common dream? If so, why? Reoccurring dreams are usually God's continual message, like life lessons that we re-encounter, until we conquer it, or live it. The dream seems to follow us, until we follow it. Common dream themes are familiar to many, and are often reoccurring. The meaning of common dream themes is provided in Addison's book.

Fourth, what are the three or four main points? While details are fascinating, too much is confusing. When we narrow it down to the main story line, we grasp the big picture that God wants us to see, like parables, short with a few main points.

After pondering these questions, consider if the dream is symbolic. Most dreams from God contain symbolism from His Word, and/or from our own environment or culture. To understand symbols, first ask what their literal meaning is, then, what would be the spiritual reflection of it? Many examples are given in Joseph's interpretations.

For example, in Pharaoh's dream, cattle symbolize years of production and years of famine. Cattle are livestock used for human consumption, and the number seven means complete (thus a complete time of production to prepare for a complete time of famine).

In the Cupbearer's dream, the three branches also represent time – three days. The vine symbolizes life (as it does in scriptures), and budding, blossoming, and ripening signify a speedy progress resulting in fruitfulness. The cup in hand means restoration of former position. This symbol is derived from the context of his life.

In the Baker's dream, there were three baskets of bread. Bread symbolizes life – nourishment, which the birds (representing Pharaoh's officers) would devour – his life. As you see, these symbols align with scriptures and the context of their lives.

God used the symbols of sand and stars in Abraham's vision, and a tree in King Nebuchadnezzar's dream. *In The Illustrated Dictionary of Dream Symbols,* author Dr. Joe Ibojie says that dreams from God come in the form of a multimedia package – full of symbols that express the mysteries of God, in parable language, or illustrated stories for His purpose:

Ultimately, God uses dreams to align our hearts, thoughts, and intentions to His eternal purpose. He may use dreams in a variety of ways: to answer our questions; to appoint us to a new mission; to command changes in the way we live; to commune with us concerning secrets of His heart; to promise us something yet to come; to teach us vital truths that we might have missed, and so forth…The message of a dream or vision can come in many ways: as prophesy, a word of knowledge; a gift of discernment; a gift of healing; a gift of wisdom…God can radically rewrite our lives through the dreams we receive. Dreams have the power to expand, confirm, enlighten, enrich, and deepen your understanding of God's word.

Dreams are personalized and specific to each individual, according to their experience and understanding. For instance, since I have had extensive study about light and darkness, I often have encouraging dreams of illumination, and dark dreams of spiritual warfare. My response is to be encouraged by the light dreams, and to pray regarding the dark dreams. As we tune into the frequency of His metaphorical language, we hear His voice more clearly and profoundly.

When Jesus communicated great spiritual concepts, he usually spoke in parables, and analogies. Though we no longer have Jesus in the flesh, we do have the "greater", Holy Spirit who teaches us through night parables, and day visions. As we move deeply into the kingdom of God, metaphorical communication brings us to a grander comprehension and perspective! God expresses His unfathomable, uncontainable concepts to those who have ears to hear, and eyes to see - speaking intimately to His children.

It may seem that we rarely hear from God in this unique way today, but it's not because He has stopped speaking in manner, for the Lord changes not. What has changed is how we may not value our dreams - by giving attention, energy, and focus to understand them. They may seem foolish to the carnal mind, because only by the Spirit of the Lord can they be understood.

The person without the Spirit does not accept the things that come from the Spirit of God but considers them foolishness, and cannot understand them because they are discerned only through the Spirit. (1 Corinthians 2:14 NIV)

As we value our dreams, our dreams will align with the values of His eternal purpose. Now let's diligently attend to His whisper.

Streaming Your Dreaming

Dreams are like mini You-tubes. Some are complete, while others are part of a series, similar to video streaming. There may be two or more parts, or layers, revealing various dimensions, or chronologies.

For instance, my husband had a two-part dream with two aspects. Part 1: A Doberman that broke through the fence to attack him. He used what was in his hand to throw at the dog, which killed the dog. The dog strangely lay dead on its back in a human form. Part 2: He saw something on the ground burning up. Here, God is showing what we see in the physical realm in part one, and what is happening in the spiritual world in part two. What was in his hand was God's Word. By streaming these parts together, we see the whole production. In the context of his life, he had recently confronted a subtle form of dark art, and which was intensely opposed.

There could be many dreams unfolding a message, purpose, or plan. Therefore, it's important to record each stream, which may be part of the whole. When we want to retain what we learn, we record in written or verbal form, as dream coach, Addison highly suggests.

Start a dream journal, with a file on your computer, phone, notebook, or verbal recording. Journal dreams, visions, symbols, clues, etc. daily no matter how insignificant it may seem. Some things are for future reference that will make sense afterwards. Include what you feel that the Lord is saying to you now. Pray that God speaks to you through His word, and notice scriptures that He brings to your attention. When you hear the whisper of the Lord accurately, note the context and how it came to you.

Become familiar with common dream themes, and biblical dream symbols, as listed in these, and many other books. Practice dream interpretation frequently for both yourself and others. The more you do, the more seasoned you will become. Ask others to write their dreams and allow you some time for interpretation. If verbal, listen attentively to the dreamer, and to God. Develop a short interpretation first, before discussing the application. You can even form a dream team, as Daniel did, with other likeminded dream interpreters. It is fun and a great outreach tool. You can also take Addison's video training online: www.dreamcrashcourse.com. What an astounding way to learn God's direction, protection, and application in your life! As we speak His language, we become more attuned to His voice, and fulfilled beyond our imagination!

Dreams indeed, reflect the supernatural world. Some dreams that we don't remember, or understand, are when the Lord is communing directly with our spirit, or our subconscious mind, and has sealed it up. He is sculpting us, just as he was shaping Job.

"Indeed God speaks once, or twice, yet no one notices it. "In a dream, a vision of the night, When sound sleep falls on men, While they slumber in their beds. Then He opens the ears of men, And seals their instruction, That He may turn man aside from his conduct, And keep man from pride" (Job 33:14-17 NASB).

Dreams and visions will become increasingly abundant and crucial as the end times are approaching. Prophesies will be our life preserver, our Lord's way of sheltering and providing for His precious bride, the church, as He preserved the whole nation and the world though Pharaoh's dream. This is where we will begin in the continuation of this book in *The Gems of Revelation,* your Wellness Preparation.

The Gems of Genesis began with valuing our sleep, and ends with cherishing our dreams. Our destination is much more than being healthy, but rather, optimum health is the vehicle that propels us to soar in our high calling. Each small step towards wholeness escorts us to full maturity, as we become the rainbow of the light of Christ, piercing through the darkness! Goodnight and God bless.

Recommended Readings:

Understanding Your Dreams Now: Spiritual Dreams Interpretation by Doug Addison
Illustrated Dictionary of Dream Symbols: A Biblical Guide to Your

Dreams and Visions by Dr. Joe Ibojie
Discovering Your Authentic Core Values: A step-by-step guide by Marc Alan Schelske

In the final chapter, we'll see why we spiritually thrive as we *fulfill* Jesus' mission in our lives.

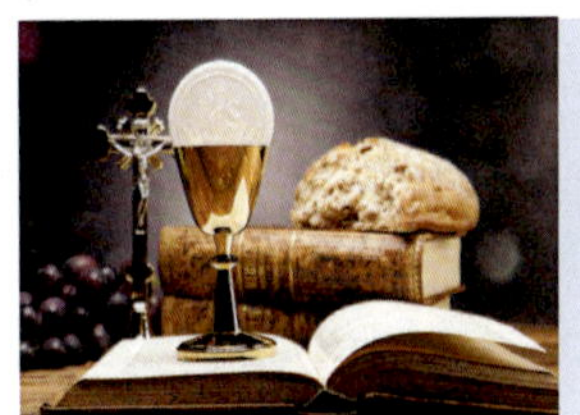

Chapter 13

Nourishing the Spirit

God's word nourishes our spirit as we read, speak, and meditate, yet it truly brings us to life when we are *giving* the Word of Life to others. We experience complete spiritual fulfillment and joy by continuing in our Lord's healing ministry.

"Jesus summoned His twelve disciples and gave them authority over unclean spirits, to cast them out, and to heal every kind of disease and every kind of sickness. "Heal the sick, raise the dead, cleanse the lepers, cast out demons. Freely you received, freely give" (Matthew 10:1,8 NASB).

By freely giving, we mature in the vine to reach out with His compassionate hands, in our time.

The Lord has given each of us His healing ministry to carry on with the power to do all that He commanded. Each disciple is *individually* named, beginning with *the first, Simon, who is called Peter.* Simon, who was once a pebble sinking in the turbulent waters became the Rock, fulfilling each command of his healing ministry, *proclaiming the kingdom, healing the sick, raising the dead, cleansing the leper, and casting out demons.*

Since these are each a part of our whole healing ministry, it's imperative that we understand how they all support our complete mission, and that we are prepared to perform, as the Lord directs.

Proclaiming the Kingdom

Jesus used many illustrations to help his followers understand what is meant by the kingdom of Heaven. He told parables that related to various walks of life to convey these spiritual truths to *everyone*. He used imagery from farming, gardening, cooking, treasure hunting, shopping, and fishing. With earthly minds trying to stretch beyond the parameters of time and place, His disciples grappled with *when* and *where* this kingdom could be. Yet Jesus portrayed the kingdom not as a *place or time*, but rather as a *relationship*—the most amazing relationship—with Him.

He tells of a man who finds a hidden treasure and a merchant who finds fine pearls, and realizing the value of what they found, they sold all else in their lives to invest in their true riches. So it is, as the classic hymn lyrics say, "Turn your eyes to Jesus, look full in his wonderful face, and the things of earth will grow strangely dim, in the light of His glory and grace."

Similarly, Jesus so *treasures* us, like priceless pearls that he gave his own life, investing all that He is, in us. He became sin for us, taking on our identity so that we could take on *His* identity. His passionate love for us yearns to *touch* every life with His healing power, for He is our Great High Priest *touched* by the feeling of our infirmities.

In another parable, Jesus tells how the enemy subtly sows a seed while everyone was sleeping, but when the Lord finally harvests, He will uproot the weeds. In this story, the servant said, "Sir, didn't you sow good seed in your field? Where then did the weeds come from?"

"An enemy did this," he replied.

Although this parable refers to the end times, it also enlightens us to our present battle, which begins as *seeds*. Seeds of disease, sickness, and dysfunction are subtly implanted by worry and fear. Then we fertilize it by giving it attention, focus, and energy, thereby using the L.O.A. *against* ourselves. And so the master rightly answers, "The enemy did this."

Jesus compares the Kingdom of Heaven to a mustard seed. This tiny seed, becomes the largest of plants, a tree of support for the birds to perch in its branches. It is this *seed* in us, where the fruit of the spirit grows bountifully, and where faith (also compared to a mustard seed) matures to receive God's abundant healing in our lives. We may not always be able to stop the enemy from sowing seeds, but we can claim God's promise that He will uproot the weeds.

Healing the Sick

When we heal the sick, our own spirit is enriched, as the Holy Spirit increases our seed of faith. When one's healing is manifest, we feel unspeakable joy. If one's healing is not immediately seen, at least we have planted a seed that can be watered. Most people are at least grateful to receive prayer, regardless of the outcome. Here are some thoughts from *street healers* and those who conduct healing sessions in a structured form.

When possible, try to establish rapport by asking the sick or injured what happened, when, etc. Share God's healing promise that He passionately yearns to heal. As you begin in prayer, invite *the Healer,* The Holy Spirit's presence, and simply follow His lead. He may give specific commands to repair, rejuvenate, or realign the body or mind. He may also give specific spiritual root causes, which we'll address in this series. He may provide general information, or His divine intervention may be *no intervention.* Such was the case with my teenage son.

He was in an accident that broke his arm, leaving his wrist bowed and front tooth bent half way back. At the emergency room, I quietly prayed for him. The attending physician said that his bone may need to be reset and oral surgery may be required for his tooth. Later, when the specialists saw him, they did nothing, but said he should see another specialist the next day. I was furious; why didn't they do something? Little did I know that the *lead* attending physician, Jesus, would heal my son in another way — naturally. The next day, the orthopedic decided to simply cast his arm, and the dentist showed him how to place his tongue as a support for re-grounding his tooth. Both healed beautifully!

Another important point is that healing occurs when we pray, not when the symptoms subside. This truth becomes reality when the sick or injured put their faith in action, like the man with the withered hand, who stretched forth his hand and the lame man who packed up his bed. Jesus often gave a specific command that allowed them to activate their faith.

Some who practice healing release spiritual energy by laying hands on the sick or anointing with oil, the symbol of the Holy Spirit penetrating, and some simply pray. Yet, what they all have in common is that they speak boldly to remove the *mountain* and speak with authority to the *roots of the fig tree.* They developed this gift of healing simply by doing it, as the Lord commanded and guided them.

Raising the Dead

Raising the dead might *raise* some big concerns. Is this really possible? Should I intervene once someone dies? Why is this included as part of our healing ministry?

Would Jesus give us a command that we couldn't fulfill? Let's look at *who* those were that Jesus, Peter, Paul, and others raised from the dead. Most were young people who had died prematurely, who had not yet fulfilled their purpose in life. Through resurrection, God restores His healing power in their lives. God raised his own son, who then *finished* the work of our redemption. Consider the promise of God:

...I will remove sickness from your midst...I will fulfill the number of your days (Exodus 23:25-26 NASB).

In *Divine Healing Made Simple*, the *Praying Medic* shares four considerations for raising the dead. First, that death is the will of the enemy, who steals, kills, and destroys. Second, that although life is God's will, we need to ask to know what His will is for that individual. This might come in the form of a dream or vision, through a word of knowledge or of wisdom, or by an angel. God will then give specific instructions for each situation. Whatever you do, you should do it confidently, like Jesus said to Jarius, (Do not be afraid; only believe, and she will be *made well.*) From Jesus' point of view, her death was a state of not *being well*, or as he called it in Lazarus' case, a state of sleep. Like healing, we need to develop confidence in God's ability and *desire* to raise the dead.

The other two considerations are for the departed, their friends, and family. Does the departed one actually want to come back once they've entered eternity? "You wouldn't want to bring someone back to life only to hear them say, OMG, why couldn't you just let me go? Did I forget something?"

The Praying Medic shares that in most cases of near-death experiences, the person was actually clinically dead and returned. He claims that about 90% who remembered the experience said that they died prematurely and had to return because it was not yet their time to die. Others reported that they were given a choice to remain in heaven or go back. Those who chose to return were granted their request. On the other hand, each of us has an appointed time of departure, and some would prefer eternity rather than returning to earth.

Finally, talking with family and friends may provide valuable insight about the individual. They may feel that the departed left prematurely, or they may see this as God's will, in which case a resurrection is unlikely and may potentially cause problems. The proper protocol would certainly be to ask the family and friends for permission. Should you have the green light, proceed with prayer—through faith, to enter boldly into the throne of the Almighty—in the powerful Name of Jesus Christ.

Considering all of this, take confidence in the command of the Lord Jesus to raise the dead.

My personal testimony involves raising animals from the dead. When I was a young teen, our family dog gave birth to several puppies out in the snow, and when my sisters found them, the babies were frozen stiff. I had just returned home from a Bible study, and I guess the Lord was starting my *on the job training* the minute I walked in. By then, the puppies had thawed, but were still lifeless. I told them to put the puppies on the rug in our bedroom. We sat encircling the puppies, and I began reading from the book of Acts. About 10 minutes later, something startling happened. A few of them began moving and came back to life!

You can read many online testimonies of people who were resurrected. At the end of the chapter, "Raising the Dead" by the Praying Medic, he shares about a Bible college in Africa where the graduation requirement for ordination is raising someone from the dead.

Cleansing the Leper

Leprosy is an infectious disease that produces sores, and can mar the skin with large, disfiguring lumps. Leprosy causes nerve and muscle damage, and may eventually lead to the loss of the use of hands and feet. The term *cleansing* the leper refers to removing the active source of the infection. Today, we don't see much leprosy, especially in northern climates, but there is certainly a big concern for many other infectious diseases. Recall in chapter two that *light* is the most powerful form of antibiotic. As we carry the spiritual light of Christ, we are called lights, and His presence in us has the power to cleanse any disease!

Casting out Demons

The root cause of some disease or illness is demonic influence, and therefore, the demon must be evicted before one is healed. There is not usually demon possession, but rather demonic influence. This is not a reflection on the victim, for we are all victims of darkness at some point, which is why we needed a savior from the very beginning. As we are engaged in our healing ministry, the Lord will help us discern specific spirits to be removed.

Deliverance ministry, however, where demonic spirits are involved, should only be performed by mature trained Christian believers. Ideally, in a neutral and positive environment where there is plenty of natural light. Indeed, this is a very sensitive form of ministry to be practiced with respect and great forbearance to prevent yourself from the evil spirit's influence. Much study and scriptural grounding are essential.

A spiritual cause is likely the culprit when there is nothing that can be found medically wrong, or no logical reason in the physical realm. Such was the case when my mother came home from rehab, recovering from hip replacement surgery. She was finally getting better when upon her second day back home, she began experiencing chronic neck pain. After numerous tests, the hospital couldn't find the source. By then, I was getting real mad at the devil. As I prayed for her, the Lord told me to rebuke the *spirit of pain*, and in that hour, the pain left.

Jesus healed a woman who had a spirit of infirmity for eighteen years. He first delivered her from this spiritual influence, *"And He laid His hands on her; and immediately she was made erect again and began glorifying God"* (Luke 13:13 NASB).

He removed the root cause first. In other healings, he spoke directly to the spirit of *deafness*, spirit of *dumbness*, and spirit of *blindness*. Notice that these are all conditions that prevent normal bodily functions.

In the scriptures, we see that spirits have certain *specialties*, and that they operate in a militaristic way. Therefore, the Lord can reveal to us their specialty, and we can speak with authority over the unclean spirit, like a sergeant demanding it to depart in the Name of Jesus Christ our Lord!

I learned to speak like this after my son adopted a pit bull named Oreo. As the dog grew, he became more and more *bullish* and would back me into a corner, barking aggressively. Finally, I was fed up, and, I strongly commanded him, "Oreo, Get Into Your Crate—NOW!" and into his crate he ran! Once I established authority, I was no longer afraid. He obeyed my persistent bold tone. God gives us the gift of discernment as we need to know how to deal with various situations.

Some time ago, I had a dream that there was an elderly woman hovering over a sick person in bed. She spoke sincerely and sweetly, "My dear, if you're sick, there's nothing you can do about it."

I woke up and asked the Lord, "What was that about?"

Then I heard the words, "A lying religious spirit." I believe that God was teaching me discernment of this spirit through my dream.

Our healing ministry is an extension of our Lord's healing ministry. It is our *Fulfillment Land.* It is the Kingdom of Heaven *living* in you, by speaking those things that appear not, yet to come into being. It is your voice of victory, and your whisper of praise. Whatever you *loose* in His kingdom will be loosed on earth, and that which you bind in His kingdom will be bound on earth – His Kingdom – on earth as it is in heaven.

May we step out of our Lord's classroom, and let *loose* His kingdom by proclaiming and *reclaiming* it. Heal the sick, raise the dead, cleanse the leper, and cast out demons!

Recommended Readings:

Christ the Healer by F.F. Bosworth

Divine Healing made Simple by Praying Medic

How to Heal the Sick by Charles and Frances Hunter

Conclusion

Great are the works of the Lord, studied by all who delight in them (Psalm 111:2 ESV).

In *The Gems of Genesis*, we have only seen a glimpse of this bountiful cornucopia of healing modalities, through darkness, lights, colors, seasons, land, water, and Adam and Eve. What an amazing display of God's love, who desires above all that we prosper and retain health through His plan for restoration in creation.

As we journey through our personal Genesis, let us embrace the gems that spark our interest and allow their brilliance to *sculpt in us* new angles that lead to lifelong fulfillment. *The Gems of Genesis* lends a fresh perspective that we can become balanced by the polarities of the universe and polished with these luminous treasures found in God's word. You can behold these marvelous gemstones in your own hands with the help of recommended books in each section and explore further by your own research. The Health Coach Recommendations can be your springboard to wellness to increase energy, endurance, and balance.

Remember, God's pharmacy is always well stocked, always open, and you won't have to take a loan out for your meds. In fact, just a few bucks can buy some of the best medicine on the planet! The health benefits of *glorious greens* rejuvenate the body and mind with vitality and creativity; *great grains* sustain a healthy heart; *fantastic fruits* cleanse and protect; *fabulous fats* invigorate all bodily systems; and *perfect proteins* spur development and healing. The *side effects* of the Lord's medicine are in bold print:

Vitality, strength, and longevity.

May we reach up and grasp our own rainbow, and use the medicinal colors to heal, by soothing pains, stimulating functions, and balancing our overall well-being. May we bask in the light, the ultimate antibiotic, and trust The Lord through our darkness into the light of new perspectives and insights.

Live your full life, fully alive! This is what F.F. Bosworth, author of *Christ the Healer*, did. When he was 81, he retired to bed early one evening and told his family that God had shown him that he had "finished his course," his ministry, and that it was time to go home. He said, "I sure don't want to hang around down here." He prayed that he would glorify God in his death as he had in his life, without sickness. As he was transitioning into eternity, his family could hear him greeting and hugging others. Occasionally, he would say, "Oh, it is so beautiful." After several hours, he put his head back and slept.

Surely, this is how our Heavenly Father intends for us to depart this life, in a peaceful, fully functional, healthy way. Yet while we are here on earth, let us adorn our earthen vessel with the crown of health bejeweled with the vibrant *Gems of Genesis*. May you live *your* full life, *fully alive!*

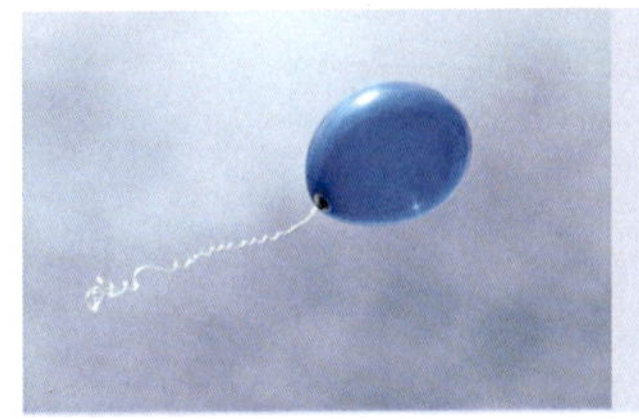

Afterword

For behold, he who forms the mountains and creates the wind, and declares to man what is his thought, who makes the morning darkness, and treads on the heights of the earth— the Lord, the God of hosts, is his name! (Amos 4:13 ESV)

The morning after I finished writing this book, I had a dream that I had cut a hole through my window screen, and released a balloon. I couldn't see the balloon as it rose to the sky, but I felt joy as it was ascending, and I knew it had a destiny. As I pondered the meaning of this brief scene, I asked the Lord what this was about. The next thoughts came to mind.

The window screen is merely fabric, yet it separates us from the real world – the outdoors. The outdoors is both literal and figurative. It is creation, where, as we have seen, emanates amazing natural and supernatural healing gems. It is also outside of the parameters of our mind, where we are not restricted to mechanical healing, but rather, harnessing the powers of our Creator. These parameters are only the fabric of our thoughts – fabricated self-limiting beliefs. I encourage you to consider cutting a hole through whatever is holding you back from fully experiencing all of the fullness of life that God has for you. I pray that this book is a refreshing guide for your journey.

The balloon represents joy. It is my great joy to break through the screen, releasing *The Gems of Genesis.* While its destination is not visible, I hope that you will catch it, and embrace these gemstones, polishing them in your own unique way that your joy may be bursting with abundant life!

Behold, the One who forms the mountains and creates the wind, who makes the morning darkness, and treads on the heights of the earth – He declares to YOU what is his thought!

About the Author

Sandy M. Stillwell is a native of Quincy, Illinois, which ironically is called the *Gem City*, due to its abundance of natural resources and trading potential. In the 1830s it was considered a "gem city."

She has lived in Maryland as a thriving entrepreneur for over 30 years. Her passion for natural health has led her to serve as a holistic, spiritual teacher, presenting *The Gems of Genesis* workshop in the Northern D.C./ Maryland area for churches, hospitals, and other organizations, and corporations. For further information, see gemsofgenesis.com.

Sandy holds a Bachelor of Arts degree in business communications and creative writing, from Quincy University. She is a certified health counselor and C.L.T. (Color Light Therapist), a graduate of the Institute of Integrative Nutrition. Her husband, Jon, two sons, Benny and Ryan, and dog, Oreo, are her strong supports.

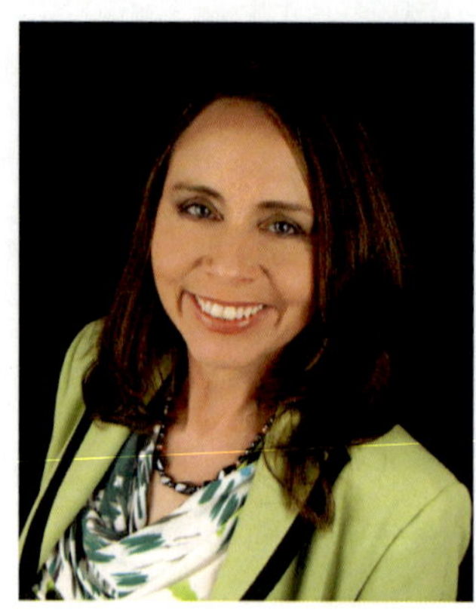